ENERGY
<u>NOW</u>

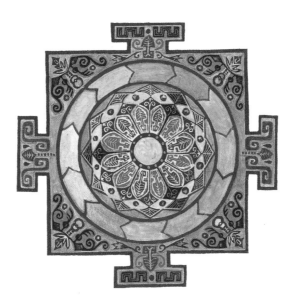

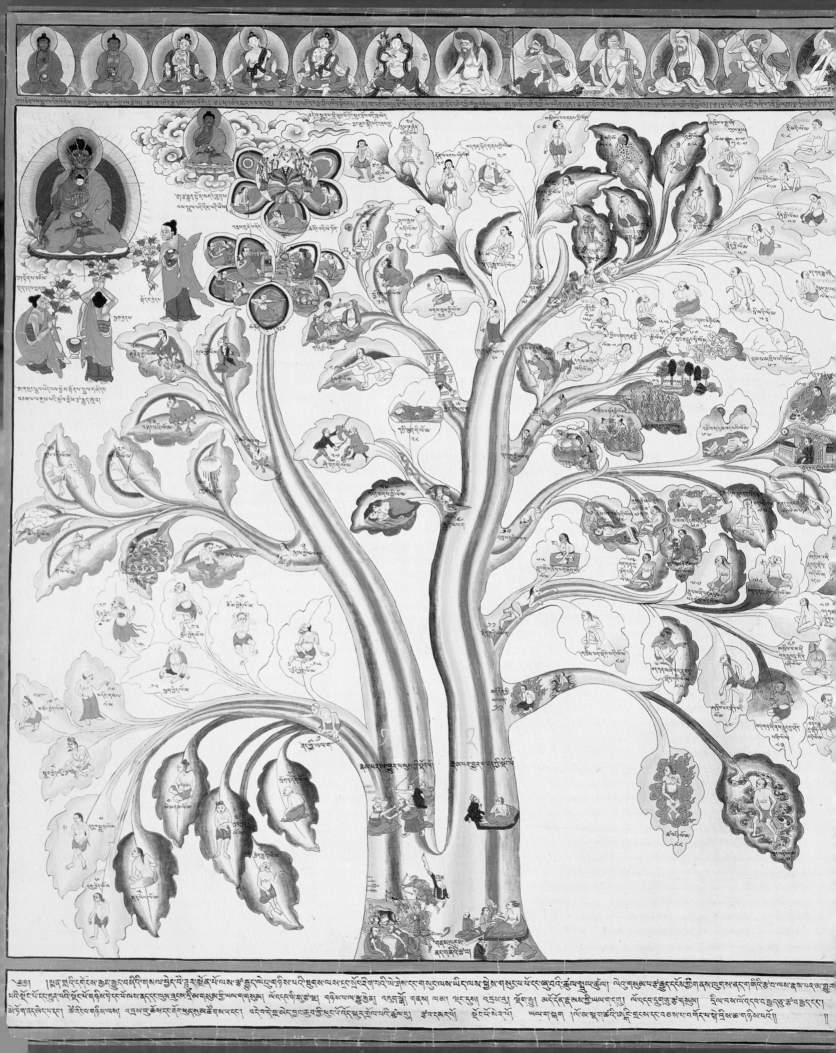

ENERGY
NOW

SIMPLE WAYS TO GAIN VITALITY,
OVERCOME TENSION, AND
ACHIEVE HARMONY AND BALANCE

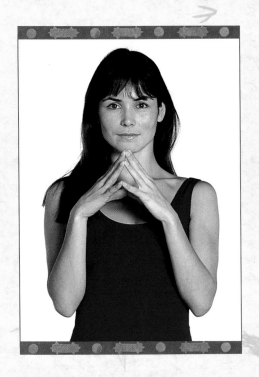

GENERAL EDITOR: EMMA MITCHELL
COMMISSIONED PHOTOGRAPHY: ANTONIA DEUTSCH

Energy Now

This edition published in 1998 by
Duncan Baird Publishers for Macmillan Publishing
USA

First published by Duncan Baird Publishers in 1998

Conceived, created, and designed by
Duncan Baird Publishers
Sixth Floor, Castle House
75–76 Wells Street
London W1P 3RE

Managing editor Catherine Bradley
Editor Slaney Begley
Designers Sue Bush, Lucie Penn
Commissioned photography Antonia Deutsch
Picture research Cecilia Weston-Baker
Principal illustrator Elaine Cox
Prop buyer Tara Solesbury
Indexer Drusilla Calvert

Library of Congress Cataloging-in-Publication Data

Energy now / general editor, Emma Mitchell
       p.   cm.
    Includes bibliographical references and index.
    ISBN 0-02-862675-3
    1. Alternative medicine.   2. Vital force—
Therapeutic use.   3. Health.   4. Vitality.   I. Mitchell,
Emma.   II. Title: Energy now.
R733.E535   1998
615.5—dc21   98-6835
                              CIP

1 3 5 7 9 10 8 6 4 2

Typeset in Garamond and Goudy
Color reproduction by Colourscan, Singapore
Printed in Singapore by
Imago Publishing Limited.

Publisher's note
Before following any advice or exercises contained in
this book, it is recommended that you consult your
doctor if you suffer from any health problems or
special conditions or are in any doubt as to its
suitability. The publishers, DBP, the authors, and the
photographer cannot accept responsibility for any
injuries or damage incurred as a result of following the
exercises in this book, or using any of the therapeutic
methods that are mentioned herein.

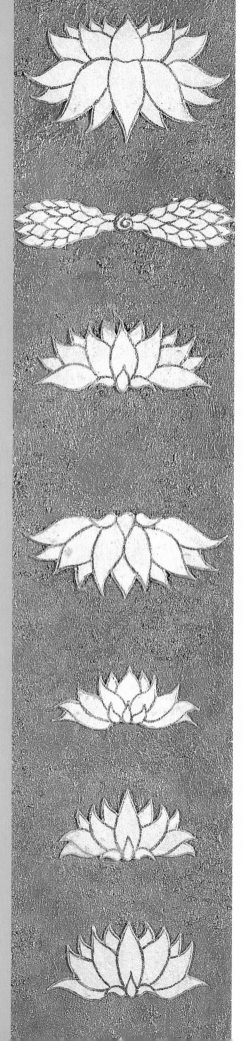

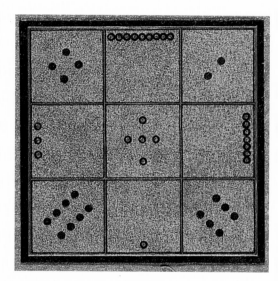

" Miracles do not happen in contradiction to nature, but only in contradiction to that which is known to us in nature. "

ST AUGUSTINE

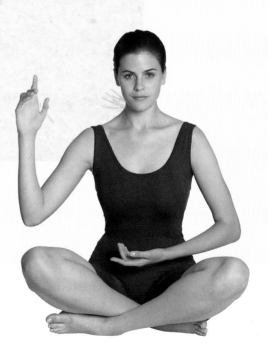

CONTENTS

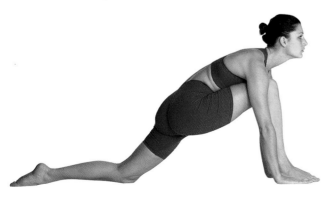
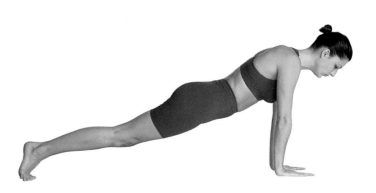

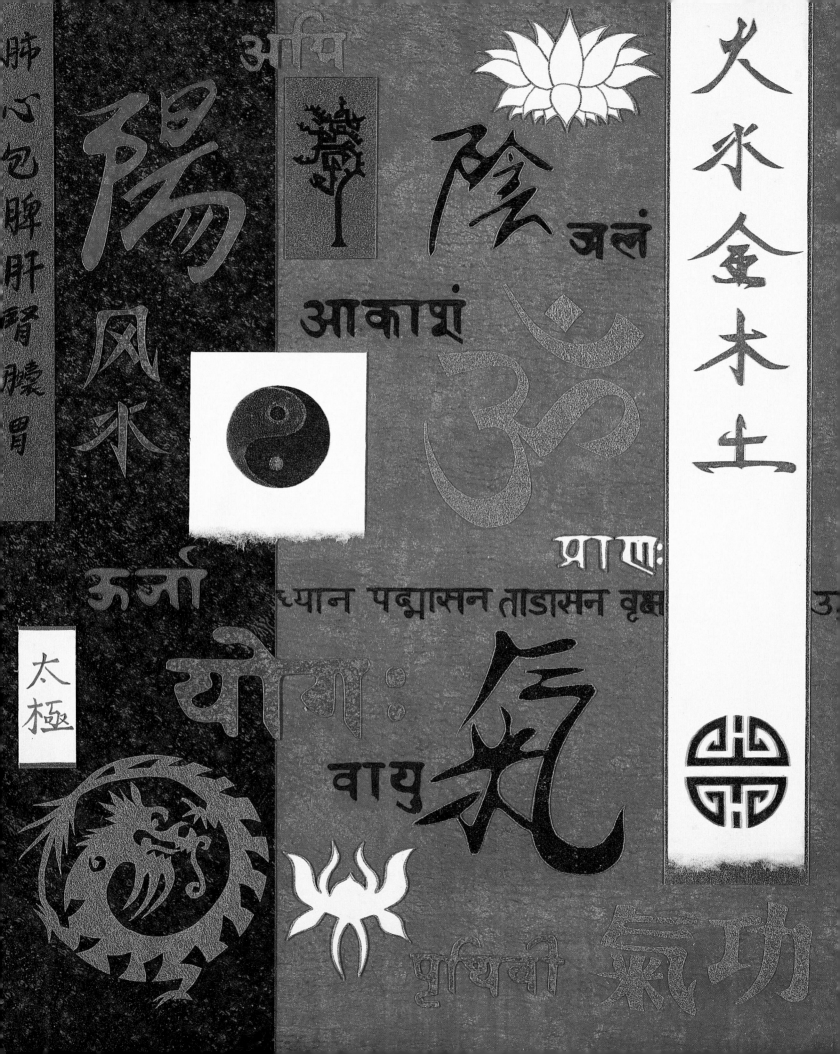

INTRODUCTION

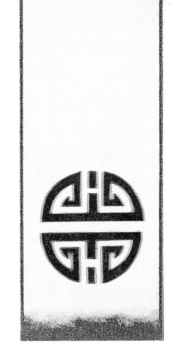

In the West, orthodox medicine envisages the body as a machine—a functioning set of working parts. In organ transplant, for example, we are now able to remove a part that is "not working" and replace it. However, many diverse cultures believe that the body is more than a collection of parts. They acknowledge an essential inner energy that is constantly flowing through the body from conception, throughout life, and perhaps into the afterlife. This energy is known in China as Qi (or Chi, pronounced "chee"), in India as Prana, and in Tibet as Lung. Although the concept now seems alien to many Western minds, it was once accepted in Europe too. The ancient Greek physician Galen called the body's energy Pneuma, and medieval alchemists used the term Vital Fluid.

Today, there are three main models that are used to explain the body's energy: the ancient Chinese system, the ancient Indian system, and the modern Western model. Each has developed independently, but shows striking similarities to the other two. According to all three systems, energy permeates the physical body—the organs, muscles, bones, and glands that we can dissect and examine—but also reaches beyond the physical into areas that Western allopathic medicine does not address. These systems define health and illness not only on the physical level, but also on the mental and spiritual planes through observing the state of the body's energy. Illness is believed to begin when the energy flow is first disrupted, rather than when physical symptoms appear. The balance of energy in the body can be deeply affected by stress, shock, or emotional factors. If the energy remains unbalanced, illness will result. Good health depends on a smooth, steady flow of energy, which requires mental and spiritual, as well as physical, balance. Each of the three main systems has evolved its own theories on medicine, exercise, nutrition, and lifestyle to achieve this.

The Chinese body energy system is so ancient that its roots cannot be traced. Its influence has been strongest in the Far East, extending south from China through Laos, Thailand, and Cambodia to the Philippines, and east through Korea to Japan. It is the foundation of Oriental Medicine, "soft" martial arts such as Qigong and T'ai Chi, and many schools of mental and spiritual development. The key concept of the Chinese system is that there are "rivers of energy," known as meridians, that run through the body. There are twelve main meridians with many minor branches, and eight vessels that may be considered as energy reservoirs. Energy flows through each of the meridians, one after the other, in a complete energy cycle. Each of the major meridians is associated with an organ, such as the heart, as well as with the muscles along its path; with emotions; and with the elements and the cycles of nature, whether times of day or the changing seasons. If the meridians become blocked, the flow of energy is disrupted, which can eventually lead to certain organs becoming depleted of energy and developing physical symptoms.

In the Indian approach, the body's energy is thought to generate from and be regulated by the chakra system. Chakras are thought of as "spinning wheels of energy." There are seven major chakras positioned down the midline of the body from the crown chakra at the top of the head to the base chakra at the base of the spine. There are also minor chakras located around the body. Each of the major chakras is associated with different organs, endocrine glands, emotions, abilities, and colors. The energy given out by the chakras creates an aura that reaches beyond the physical body and forms layers around the body. This body energy system is the basis of both Yoga and the Ayurvedic medical tradition and is the model followed by both Hindus and Buddhists during meditation.

The third body energy system was developed in the West and is used by healers and clairvoyants in Europe and the United States. It is similar to the Indian chakra system, in that layers of energy are believed to surround the body. These layers are linked to the chakras and form an aura. People who can see this aura describe seven distinct layers, each possessing a different color, density, fluidity, and function. The successive layers emit different "vibrations" of energy; each layer encompasses the physical body and all the previous layers, as well as reaching beyond to a more expansive energy field. Each layer is also associated with a chakra. The first layer is linked to the base or first chakra, the second to the sacral or second chakra, and so on to the seventh layer, which is associated with the crown chakra. The first three layers represent the energy of the physical being. The fourth

reflects the astral body, which is connected to the heart chakra and is associated with love. The three highest layers are the energy vibrations of the spiritual plane.

The energy within every person directly or indirectly affects the energy of every other person in the world. Our relationships with those closest to us are crucial to our well-being and happiness. We are profoundly affected by the atmosphere created by the energy of our partners, parents, children, or close friends and respond to whether they are excited, happy, or depressed. Even strangers can affect our energy—squeezing past crowds of tired and preoccupied people in a city street, for example, can be disturbing to our energy, while enjoying a concert or party surrounded by congenial people can gloriously uplift our energy. Energy moves between people via thought and meditation. It also moves through vision: we

Kirlian photographs record the energy that is emitted from every part of our bodies in the form of electromagnetic discharge. The example below is of an ordinary fingertip.

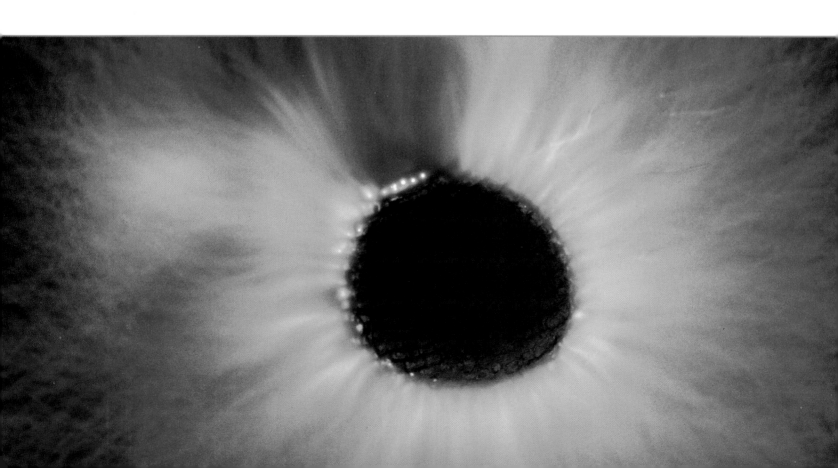

have all experienced the feeling that someone is looking at the back of our heads—a feeling arising from an innate awareness that their energy is affecting us. However, if when you turn around he or she averts their eyes, the energy link between you is broken. Energy levels vary between people. Some radiate energy and are

said to have presence. Others may pass unnoticed in a large gathering. It may be that some people possess the power to draw their energy in upon themselves, to make themselves invisible; others are able to project their energy to heal or influence people.

Most of us are not able to see each other's energy, but instinctively possess a sense of our own field—and may notice it when someone comes too close and invades our space, or when we hug a loved one. This book will help you recognize and channel your body's energy.

We are used to thinking that a healthy person is someone who is not sick or suffering. However, health is more than that—a truly healthy person is one whose energy and vitality enable him or her to fight illness. Medicine should not only be about eradicating disease, but should also strengthen our immune systems so that we can fully recover from—or successfully resist—illness.

Preventative medicine aims to keep the body healthy, strong, and well. In the West you go to an orthodox doctor when you have physical symptoms of ill health. In China, by contrast, you visit your doctor or teacher to

Exercises designed to increase the body's vital energy are practiced daily by millions of people in the East. Children from a Chinese middle school are shown above performing their morning exercises in Beijing.

In many medical traditions, the smooth flow of vital energy through the body is as important as breathing or having a pulse. This Indian doctor (right) is pointing to a chart that shows access points to the body's energy system.

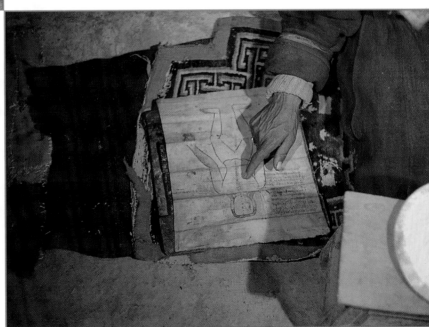

remain well. The Chinese say that treating a person when they have become ill is like starting to dig a well when you are thirsty—by that time it may be too late. Many believe that if you ensure that the energy in and around your body is flowing smoothly—that it is cleansed, refined, and in balance—then you will not become ill. Every complementary medicine, from Acupuncture to Reflexology, Ayurvedic medicine to Therapeutic Touch, uses the body's energy as its basic tool. These preventative medicines are described in this book.

Modern lifestyles can be highly stressful. Unreasonable efforts are often expected of us at work, we may live in polluted cities, exercise insufficiently, and fail to clear our minds for the deep sleep needed to recharge our depleted energy. We travel in airplanes across the world, launching ourselves into different environments and time zones, a process that disrupts our natural rhythms. Computers, power stations, cables, televisions, mobile phones, and all our electronic gadgetry give out electromagnetic radiation, which disrupts our own body's energy. We have an instinctive fight-or-flight mechanism that helped our earliest ancestors when they were being attacked by wild animals. However, modern stresses rarely require us to fight or flee, but rather to sit at a desk and react with our minds while bottling up our emotions. Because it is not acceptable to react physically, this natural fight-or-flight reaction becomes repressed within us, causing stress that may block energy flow. By being more aware of your body's energy—and of the many stresses that reduce it—you can begin to achieve mental and spiritual balance and prevent illness.

Energy Now explores the widespread belief in a universal energy, and examines how you can alleviate the problems of modern living through exercise, meditation, and diet. Many people in the world have grown up with an awareness of their body's energy because it is at the root of their culture, spiritual development, and medicine. In the West it remains an unusual concept: it may be

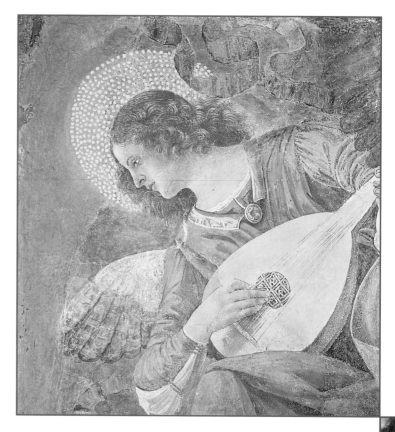

Haloes are images of the body's aura, used to symbolize holiness in paintings such as Angel Musician *by Melozzo da Forlì (1438–94).*

something that you know a great deal about, but have never put into words. You are probably already familiar with such practices as Aromatherapy and Acupuncture—this book illustrates how all of these "alternative" or "complementary" methods are based on the concept of the body's energy.

The first chapter of this book covers the Chinese and Japanese ideas of energy and also suggests some simple exercises, based on the disciplines of Qigong, Do-in, and Shiatsu, which will help you to become aware of your energy and improve the flow of this energy. The second chapter outlines how energy is perceived in the Indian tradition. It includes a series of Hatha Yoga exercises that have been designed for beginners to improve the flow of energy through their chakras.

The third chapter is about energy, posture, and movement. By being aware of our body's energy we can use it more efficiently and with great benefit in everyday activities, such as walking and sitting at a desk. Good use of the body enables the energy to flow smoothly and unimpeded through the body. Therapies that concentrate on balanced posture are introduced, such as Osteopathy, Chiropractic, Cranial Osteopathy, Craniosacral Therapy, and the Alexander Technique. The chapter also includes straightforward exercises from Qigong, T'ai Chi, Yoga, and Kinesiology for you to try.

Massage is a way of directing and smoothing the flow of the body's energy, and this is covered in the fourth chapter. There are also notes on Aromatherapy oils that affect energy and an introduction to Reflexology and pleasurable foot massage. Energy is the essential medium

Nurturing our body's energy can help us to remain healthy or to overcome illness. It may also improve our personal happiness.

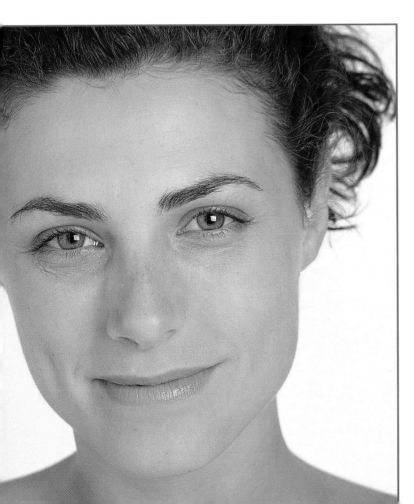

of healers, and chapter five explains some healing techniques from Acupressure, Kinesiology, and Therapeutic Touch. It also provides an introduction to Homeopathy, Ayurveda, and Chinese Traditional Medicine.

The chapter on Energy, Diet, and Living Well is full of practical tips on how you can improve the energy in your everyday life. It examines Eastern diets and methods of relaxation, and offers advice on getting a good night's sleep and relieving or reducing stress in your life. An introduction to the Chinese science of Feng Shui explains how to cleanse and direct the energy in your office and at home so that it works positively with you.

We obtain energy for life from food, clean water, fresh air, exercise, and sleep. These are things we enjoy every day and just by being aware of them we can be healthier and happier. You can gain benefit from this book at whatever level suits you. It may be most useful as a reference and introduction to the many therapies and disciplines available to you. You may choose to take advantage of the tips to improve the energy surrounding you at home or at work. As you find that small changes benefit your life, you may eventually use this book as a holistic guide for health and good living.

Energy Now is not an exercise program—you do not have to do every exercise or subject yourself to a long and arduous routine. The exercises do not form a sequence, and I suggest that you try those that appeal to you—see how they make you feel, and if they benefit you, adopt them at a time of day when they can fit easily into your life. You may enjoy a five-minute Qigong exercise first thing in the morning, or prefer to carry out the classic Yogic exercise, Saluting the Sun. You may find that the most convenient time to balance your energy is at your desk in the day or that adopting a relaxation technique in the evening gives you a more refreshing night's sleep. Try to do at least one suggested exercise for a few minutes each day, and, whatever your age and state of health, I am confident that you will notice the benefit and will soon be dipping back into this book for more.

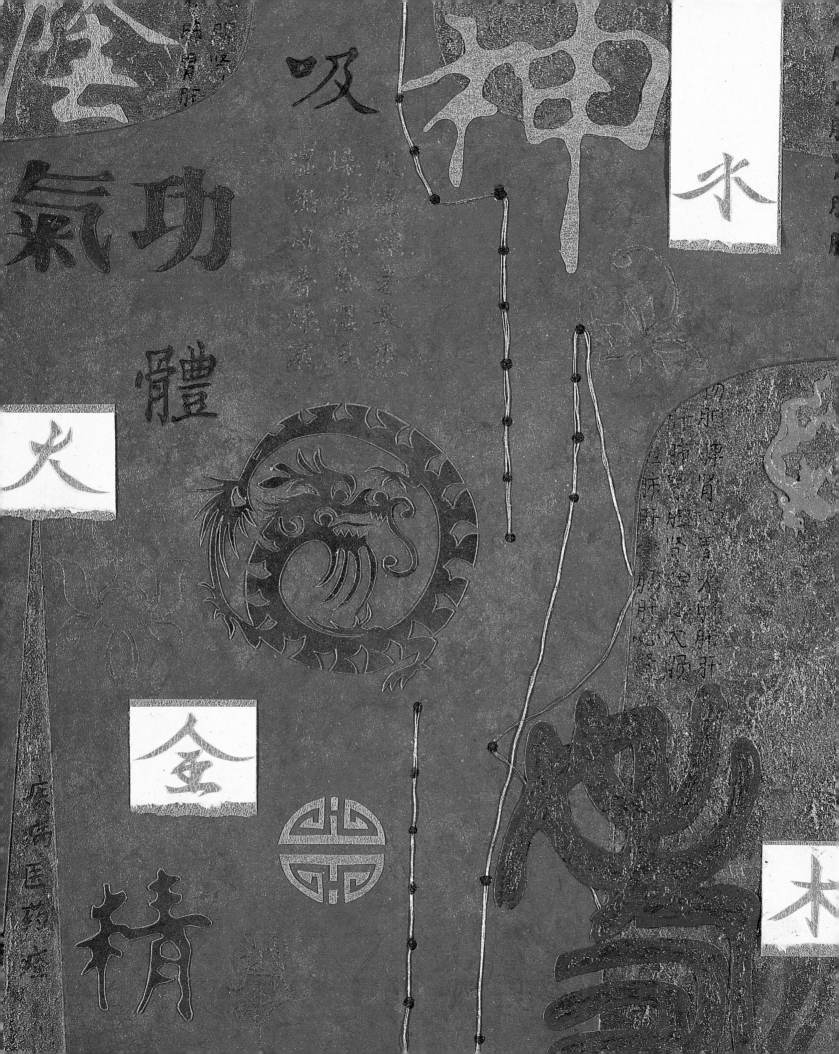

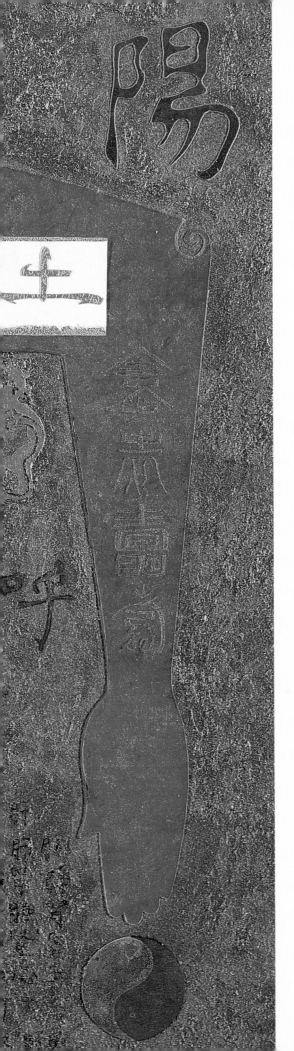

CHINESE IDEAS OF ENERGY

The energy systems of China and Japan see the body as a reflection of the universe, influenced by environmental, climatic, dietary, mental, and spiritual factors. If a person lives in harmony with the environment, he or she will be healthy, calm, and have spiritual strength. Conversely, going against the forces of nature is thought to lead to imbalance and disease.

In the Chinese system, Qi (energy) is thought to come from one universal source and is divided into two relative yet opposing forces: Yin and Yang. These forces are influenced by five elements that make up all living things. Physical and mental exercises can be used to balance the elements in the human body and to regulate the flow of Qi. Today, such exercises are practiced widely in the forms of Qigong, T'ai Chi, and other martial arts.

THE CHINESE CONCEPT OF QI

Vitality and health are determined by a good intake and balance of Qi, or vital energy, in the body. This Qi, or Chi (pronounced "chee"), is said to be not only earthly and material, but also heavenly and immaterial. Qi forms the basis of every human being's physical health and is also essential to our mental and emotional balance.

There are many different types of Qi, including Congenital Qi, Nutritive Qi, and Protective Qi. Congenital Qi, received from both parents at conception, forms the basis of one's genetic make-up. In the womb further Congenital Qi is received from the mother via the placenta. Congenital Qi, which is stored in a person's kidneys, determines levels of vitality; it may be depleted by stress, long working hours, and the intake of stimulants—

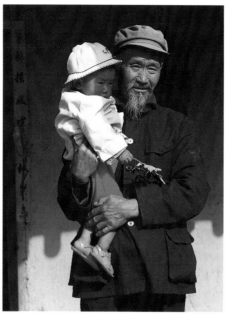

The amount of Congenital Qi in the body gradually diminishes over an individual's lifetime. Its decrease is reflected in the natural, physical signs of aging, such as graying hair and wrinkles. This process can be slowed down, however, by taking good care of the body's Qi in earlier life.

to all the vital organs. In general, foods that are high in energy have been naturally grown and freshly picked, and are eaten raw or lightly cooked. If food is re-heated, over-cooked, or filled with artificial flavorings and preservatives, it will contain little or no Qi.

Qi in air and in food is combined with bodily fluids and other substances to provide energy to all the internal organs. Another type of Qi, known as Protective Qi, surrounds the body, helping to regulate temperature and protect against cold, heat, and damp. It is also related to disease immunity and resistance.

In the Chinese system, mental energy is housed in the heart, while emotions are linked primarily to the digestive system. If a person suffers stress and emotional upset, this will disturb the heart function and cause

such as coffee, tea, and carbonated drinks. The best way to conserve vital energy is to work and sleep regular hours and to drink plenty of fresh water every day. Feelings of tiredness, enervation, or exhaustion can be indications of a deficiency of Congenital Qi.

Qi enters the body in two other main ways: the air we breathe and the food we eat. When we inhale, air enters our lungs, providing the body with Qi. Deep breathing and a regular intake of fresh air are essential to ensure a potent supply of healthy Qi within the lungs. Unfortunately, many people have poor breathing habits, exercise rarely, and inhabit environments with little or no fresh air. As a result, the body becomes weaker and more susceptible to colds and flu.

Energy from food (Nutritive Qi) is released in the stomach and is transformed by the spleen and delivered

digestive problems. Tranquil thoughts and calm analysis of situations, along with relaxed eating habits, will strengthen mental Qi and keep the emotions balanced. An inadequate supply of Qi, which often occurs through breathing polluted air, eating processed or poor-quality food, and leading a generally stressful lifestyle, is thought to be the root of many illnesses. All Chinese medicines, dietary practices, and martial arts, therefore, seek to increase the intake of healthy Qi and to ensure that it is stored and used wisely in the body.

If the body's Qi is carefully nurtured and conserved, good health and mental clarity can be maintained throughout old age. The ancient Daoist masters also believed that an abundance of Qi was the secret of longevity and would nourish their vital energy through the performance of breathing and sexual exercises.

THE ROLE OF QI, BLOOD, AND FLUIDS IN THE BODY

The spleen, kidneys, lungs, heart, and liver are responsible for transforming Qi in the body, and for distributing and regulating its flow in the meridians (see pages 18–19). These five organs are nourished and moistened by the body's blood and fluids, both of which also contain Qi.

KIDNEYS

The kidneys store the body's Congenital Qi, which stems directly from the Essence of Life or Jing. Congenital Qi is inherited genetically from one's parents and is generally of fixed quantity and quality from birth. It diminishes over the course of one's life. Because it is difficult to replenish the levels of Congenital Qi in the body, care should be taken to conserve them. Avoid overindulgence in drink, food, or sex, or the problems created by excessive work.

BODILY FLUIDS

Bodily fluids, such as saliva, digestive juices, sweat, and spinal fluids, are also influenced by the nutrients in food and drink and levels of Qi. "Clean" fluids are transported to the lungs and then dispersed around the body. They provide moisture, lubrication, and nourishment. "Dirty" fluids are excreted by the bladder and bowels.

LUNGS

The amount of Qi to be found in the lungs depends upon the cleanliness of the air and the amount of oxygen brought into the lungs. A low quantity of Qi in the lungs can contribute to colds and viral disorders, poor circulation, and tiredness. City dwellers and those working regularly in stuffy environments are particularly prone to an insufficiency of Qi in the lungs, which breathing exercises and relaxation techniques will help to redress.

SPLEEN

In Chinese medicine the spleen holds a position of great importance and plays an essential role in many vital functions, including digestion, menstruation, and even mood control. The health of the spleen and stomach depends upon the quality of food a person consumes and their eating habits. If the food is rich in Qi, then digestion will be good, and this will promote the health of the five organs.

BLOOD

Blood contains Nutritive and Congenital Qi. The two are combined in the heart, which then circulates the blood. The liver is also important, as it acts as a store for the blood when the body is resting. Blood nourishes the growth and renewal of organs and tissues. It also helps the heart to house the mind and consciousness.

MERIDIANS: THE RIVERS OF ENERGY

Qi flows along a network of channels in the body, known as meridians. Although these channels are not visible, they can be measured elecfrically and are thought to be located just below the skin.

There are 12 major meridians, most of which correspond to an organ in the body. The Qi flows in a particular direction along the meridian and follows a set cycle, starting at the lungs and ending at the liver (see arrows in the key on page 19). In this way, energy circulates along all the meridians and to all the internal organs and passes from the outside of the body to the interior and then out again.

When a person is healthy, an abundant supply of Qi flows through all the meridians in the right direction. If the flow becomes blocked or unruly, disease will follow. Such blocks must be removed for good health to return.

This late 19th-century Japanese netsuke (ivory carving) shows a physician taking pulses on the wrist of his patient.

Along each of the meridians are specific places, known as acupoints, which can be used to regulate the flow of Qi in the channel. This can be achieved by using fingertip pressure or by using needles as in Acupuncture. Exercises can also be used to regulate the flow of Qi, such as the Qigong exercises that appear on pages 24–31.

If there is inadequate Qi in a meridian, weaknesses will manifest in its related organ. For example, a poor flow of Qi in the lung meridian can lead to breathlessness. Too much Qi in a meridian, however, leads to an organ over-functioning and is often associated with pain and inflammation. The burning pain and increased urinary frequency associated with the bladder infection cystitis can be a sign of an over-functioning urinary bladder meridian.

PULSE POINTS ON THE WRIST

The amount of Qi flowing through a meridian can be determined by taking the pulse. In the Chinese system there are 12 pulses, one for each of the major meridians. There are six pulses located on each wrist, three superficial and three deep. The fingers are placed in particular positions on the wrists and the response measured both on the skin surface and deeper down in the skin tissues by applying gentle pressure. If there is a good flow of Qi, the response is regular and vibrant. If there is insufficient Qi, the response will be weak and hard to locate. If there is too much Qi, the pulse will be too full and strong.

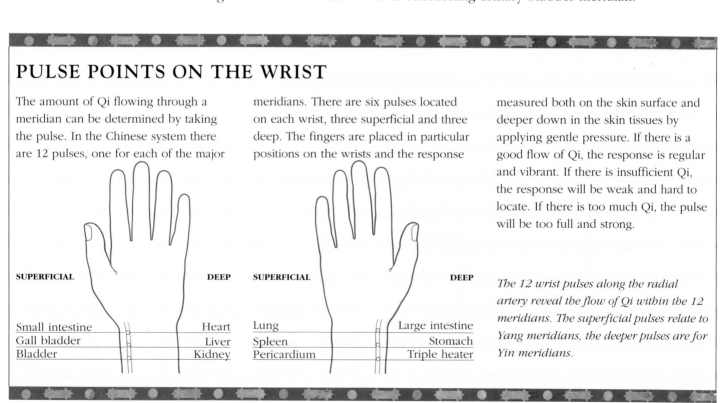

SUPERFICIAL	DEEP	SUPERFICIAL	DEEP
Small intestine	Heart	Lung	Large intestine
Gall bladder	Liver	Spleen	Stomach
Bladder	Kidney	Pericardium	Triple heater

The 12 wrist pulses along the radial artery reveal the flow of Qi within the 12 meridians. The superficial pulses relate to Yang meridians, the deeper pulses are for Yin meridians.

THE MERIDIAN NETWORK

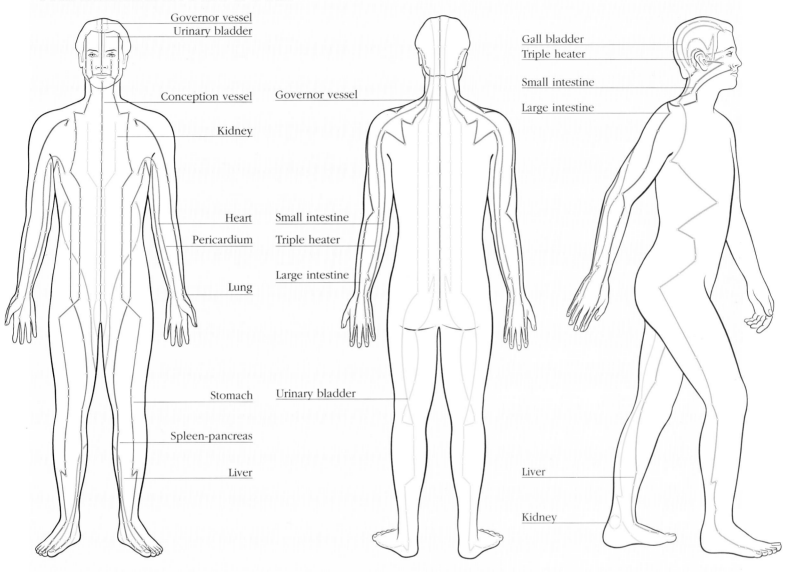

Governor vessel
Urinary bladder
Conception vessel
Kidney
Heart
Pericardium
Lung
Stomach
Spleen-pancreas
Liver

Governor vessel
Small intestine
Triple heater
Large intestine
Urinary bladder

Gall bladder
Triple heater
Small intestine
Large intestine
Liver
Kidney

Each meridian has a channel on either side of the body. The meridians function in pairs of one Yang and one Yin meridian (see right). Yang energy comes from the Sun and flows from the fingers down the face and body. Yang meridians are the large intestine, stomach, small intestine, bladder, triple heater, and gall bladder. The Qi in the Yin meridians flows from the Earth up the body and face to the fingertips. Yin meridians are the lung, spleen, heart, kidney, pericardium, and liver. The governor and conception vessels are single-channeled reservoirs of energy.

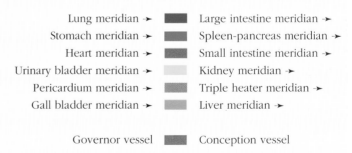

Lung meridian ➤	Large intestine meridian ➤
Stomach meridian ➤	Spleen-pancreas meridian ➤
Heart meridian ➤	Small intestine meridian ➤
Urinary bladder meridian ➤	Kidney meridian ➤
Pericardium meridian ➤	Triple heater meridian ➤
Gall bladder meridian ➤	Liver meridian ➤
Governor vessel	Conception vessel

YIN AND YANG

Qi energy manifests in both the body and the universe in the form of two complementary yet opposing forces, which are termed Yin and Yang. These two forces represent the dynamic interplay that makes up the finely balanced whole. For example, we cannot have light without dark or day without night. Yin and Yang are in constant motion, and where Yin is greatest, Yang is least. As Yin declines, Yang grows.

The theory of Yin and Yang, and the various patterns of existence that it gave birth to, was elaborated in the ancient Chinese book of divination, the *Book of Changes* (*Yi Jing* or *I Ching*). In this compendium Yang, the male principle, was represented by a continuous line, and Yin, the female principle, by a broken line. These lines were grouped in eight trigrams (combinations of three) that symbolized all the basic permutations

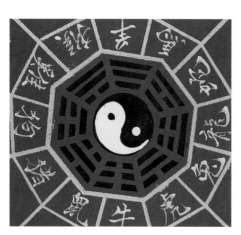

In the Great Polarity, energy (Qi) in its original form is represented as a circle, containing the dynamic forces of Yin and Yang in black and white. The eight trigrams of the Book of Changes *surround the symbol.*

of natural forces and phenomena. Traditionally, the eight trigrams were thought of as a family. Three Yang lines together represented the father, or Heaven—the Yang archetype of the creative, active principle. Three Yin lines represented the mother, or Earth—the Yin archetype of the receptive, passive principle. The six children of the family (three daughters and three sons) are known as Lake, Fire, Thunder, Wind, Water, and Mountain. Each of the eight trigrams also corresponds to a direction of the compass and a time of year, and together they represent all the fundamental states of existence to be found in the cosmos.

Yin and Yang are relative forces and cannot exist without each other. This interdependence is illustrated in the Great Polarity symbol by a seed of black in the white area, and vice versa. All things have both a Yin and a

THE FIVE ELEMENTS

Yin and Yang are further represented in the five elements that the Chinese believe make up all forms of life. These five elements—water, wood, fire, earth, and metal—also interact with each other in a dynamic cycle of support and opposition. Water can support wood, as seen in water helping trees to grow, but can destroy and quench fire.

The five elements are associated with the seasons of the year, colors, internal organs, tastes, and even emotions. Wood, for example, is linked to spring, the color green, the liver, sour tastes, and anger.

Human Qi can be divided according to the five elements and used to understand both health and disease. If someone has too much wood energy, he or she will be irascible and be prone to liver disease, while someone with insufficient water will have dry skin and hot palms and feet. A good balance of the five elements means good health and mental harmony.

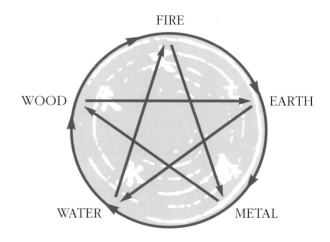

In this diagram the outer arrows depict the creative sequence of five element theory (water feeds wood feeds fire). The inner arrows show the controlling sequence (water controls fire melts metal).

Yang aspect and can be further subdivided according to Yin and Yang. For example, time can be divided into day (Yang) and night (Yin), but day can then be subdivided into morning (Yang) and afternoon (Yin). Similarly, the Moon is Yin, but moonlight is considered Yang when compared to the surrounding darkness of the night.

Yin and Yang are associated with particular qualities and manifested throughout the cosmos. Yin is associated with the feminine and with darkness, storing, inward movement, and cold. It appears in the natural world in the Moon and water and is present in the blood and interior of the body. Yang is associated with the masculine and with light, activity, external movement, and heat. In the natural world Yang is represented in the Sun and fire, and in the body it is linked to the flow of vital energy (Qi) and the external surfaces.

CHINESE PHASES AND CYCLES

According to Yin-Yang theory, all the world's energies are interrelated and in a constant state of flux. This explains the rotation of the seasons and the daily passage of the Sun through the heavens. Midwinter and midnight are considered to be highly Yin and each is followed by an increase in Yang energy, manifesting itself in qualities such as warmth and light, until Midsummer and midday, which are almost pure Yang. From this moment there is an increase in cold, dark Yin energy, while the strength of Yang energy begins to wane.

Our bodies are also governed by Yin and Yang, so it is important that we live in harmony, rather than in conflict, with the natural energies of the world. This includes adapting our levels of activity to the season and eating food that has the right qualities for our constitution.

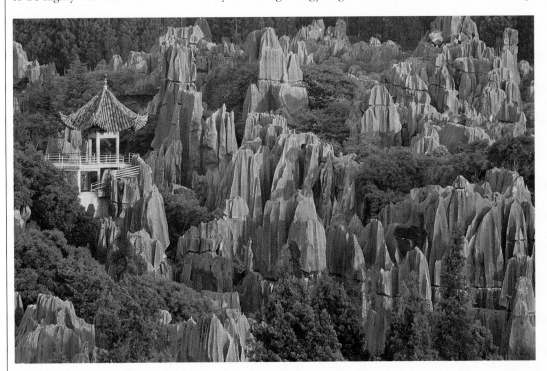

Landscapes can be analyzed in terms of the Yin-Yang and five element theories. As in all things, the balance of their energies changes with the time of day, the month, and the season. However, they also have fundamental characteristics. Rocks, such as this limestone formation in Yunnan, Kunming, China, are a powerful, and often disruptive, form of metal energy, which has here been channeled upward by the triangular-roofed building.

INTRODUCING QIGONG

The name Qigong consists of two Chinese words: Qi and Gong. Qi refers to the subtle energy that gives the physical body life and vitality. In other words, if we see every living being as the offspring of Great Nature, Qi is the force that connects human beings to Nature.

Gong, the second half of Qigong, means repeated time and labor. A calligrapher who writes with their brush day after day is practicing Bi (brush) Gong. A martial arts expert's repetition of simple punching and kicking actions is called Wu (martial) Gong. Daoist practitioners who try to harmonize Yin and Yang energy through sexual intercourse call it Bedroom Gong. Spending time drinking and appreciating tea is called Gong Fu Tea. Here in the West it might be as easy to find people who are devotees of Gong Fu Coffee. On one level, therefore, Qigong means repeated energy work or exercise.

Qigong and its precursors have a long tradition in China—there are records showing that over 5,000 years ago people were imitating animal movements to ward off cold and damp in the winter. Over the years Qigong has been developed and refined by Buddhist, Confucian and Daoist scholars, indigenous doctors, and martial arts practitioners. Today, around 60 million Chinese use it as a way of healing and maintaining good health, and it is becoming increasingly accepted in the Western world.

Qigong has two basic features: subtle and internal. It is subtle because the nature of Qi is non-physical and insubstantial. It is internal because we are focusing our energy within ourselves. It requires a concept of seeing that is different from our ordinary perception. Practicing Qigong needs a lot of careful attention and sensitivity.

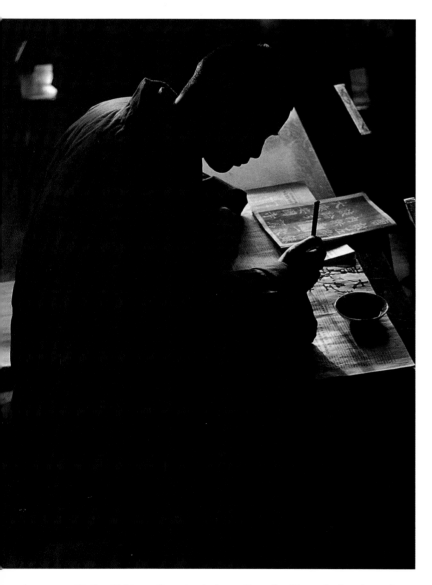

To the Chinese, the repeated practice of calligraphy brush strokes is known as Bi Gong. This monk is seen perfecting his art at the Buddhist temple of Fayuan Si in Beijing.

LI BAI AND THE OLD WOMAN

The concept of Gong is difficult for many people in the West to comprehend. A simple illustration is given in the following Chinese story.

When he was a little boy, Li Bai did not apply himself to his studies but spent his time at play. One day he met an old woman by a river rubbing a big iron bar. He became curious and asked the old woman what she was doing. "I am making a needle," she replied. "How can you possibly make a needle out of this huge iron bar?" Li Bai was amused by the idea. "Well, if one devotes enough Gong the iron bar can be made into a needle." Li Bai was so inspired by the woman's enormous determination that he vowed to study diligently. He eventually became one of the greatest poets in Chinese history.

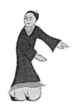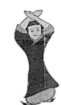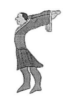

Dedicated practitioners must perform Qigong for hours every day to maintain their energy levels and skills. To practice once for several hours is easy. To practise several hours a day for several weeks is not that difficult. But to practice many hours every day for many years is another matter.

The basic methods in which Qigong develops the body's energy can be divided into four categories: body positioning, energetic movements, breathing, and meditation. Qigong includes standing, sitting, and lying down positions to help open and unify the body. Energetic movements, such as shaking, turning, stretching, rubbing, slapping, and pushing, aid synchronization and coordination. Observing the quality of your breathing may encourage it to become deep, smooth, slow, and quiet. Meditation both relaxes the body and rests the mind.

Many different styles and schools of Qigong have developed over the years, such as Buddhist (Qi) Gong, Daoist (Qi) Gong, Medical (Qi) Gong, and Martial Gong. The most widely practiced schools in China are Fragrance (Qi) Gong, Flying Crane Gong, Mind Moving Gong, and Middle Way Gong.

The Qigong exercises in this book were developed by Zhixing Wang, who teaches a style known as Hua Gong. This is particularly concerned with health, self-healing, fitness, clarity, and spiritual realization. Hua

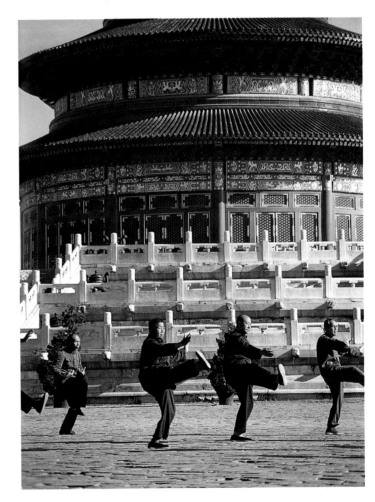

This detail from the Daoyin Xing Qi Fa, *a silk book from c. 168* B.C.E., *shows a man doing an energy exercise.*

means transformation—"Hua Gong is like a rainbow appearing"—and if you practice Hua Gong diligently and with an open mind you should experience an inner transformation. For some people the change is very fast—it is not unusual for someone to feel a vast improvement in their state of mind after a single weekend course of Hua Gong.

The following exercises are given as an introduction to Hua Gong, but it is always advisable for beginners to start in a class. Women who are pregnant are recommended not to practice unless under expert supervision.

Today, many people practice Qigong, T'ai Chi, or other forms of exercise in China to strengthen their body's energy. This photograph was taken outside the Temple of Heaven in Beijing.

SENSING THE QI

The concept of Qi is very subtle and is not easily explained using words. The best way to appreciate Qi is to feel it for yourself. Ideally, you should search out a Qigong Master who will initiate you and help you to gain a sense of your own inner energy. However, you can try the following exercises, which will help you to feel the Qi between your own hands, and to balance and strengthen the flow of Qi throughout your body. Qigong uses various postures and movements, which act like keys to open up or "plug in" to the wider energy of the universe. Once you have made that contact, the Qi within your body should move naturally, so that the exercises become very easy, light and enjoyable. Some people feel the Qi easily; others do not. If you have difficulty in making the contact do not be discouraged. Remember that for centuries people have felt and benefitted from Qigong. You can too: if you have the patience and tenacity, your efforts will be greatly rewarded.

Select one or two of the following exercises and practice them every day. When you have finished your practice, shake your whole body. Gently tap all over your head and slap down your limbs and trunk lightly. Concentrate on your feet, shaking them for a couple of minutes, then lightly run on the spot, making sure that you are aware of the Earth. Give yourself a final shake all over and feel your mind clear and refreshed.

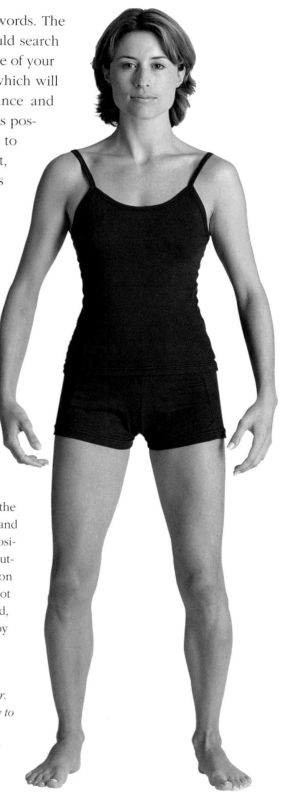

BASIC POSTURE

Many Qigong exercises begin in the basic posture, which is designed to ease the flow of Qi through your body. Your feet should feel connected with the Earth, and your head and body should be relaxed and aligned. You can meditate in this position for as long as you like. You may find it easier to look inward, rather than outside yourself, if you have your eyes closed. Forget everything that is going on around you, empty your mind and feel that you are just being; that you are not doing anything at all except standing still. You should feel as if time has stopped, that all your worries and troubles have melted away. Let your mind rest and enjoy the feelings of peace, stillness and tranquility.

Stand with your feet parallel and a shoulders' width apart. Bend your knees and gently draw up your abdominal muscles so that your behind sinks toward the floor. Keep your head erect, as if it is being held from above, and drop your chin slightly to relax your neck and face.

Lower your shoulders and allow your arms to hang loosely by your sides, so that air can circulate under your armpits. Relax completely, as if your center of gravity is pulling you deep into the Earth, yet your body feels light and alert.

SENSING A BALL OF ENERGY BETWEEN YOUR HANDS

This exercise will help you to feel a concentration of energy between your hands. The more you practice it, the more easily you should be able to feel the Qi. If at first you are not too sure whether you can feel it or not, keep going: the energy will build up and intensify. Your fingers may tingle, you may find your hands become warm, or you may feel as if you are holding something. With practice, the moment you place your hands in this position you will be able to feel the energy between your hands. At the same time you may experience the sensation that the ball of energy is also within your abdomen, emanating from the Chinese energy center known as the lower dantien.

The lower dantien is the area just below the navel—around three fingers' width down—deep inside the body almost to the spine. The exact position varies with different people. In Chinese tradition, this is the seat of our being. It is sometimes known as the "fiery furnace," because it is believed that it is from this point that our vital energy is kindled. The lower dantien needs to be stoked up regularly using exercises such as the one outlined below.

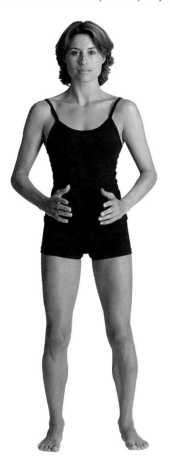

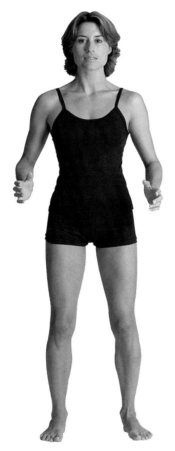

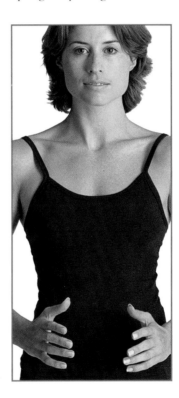

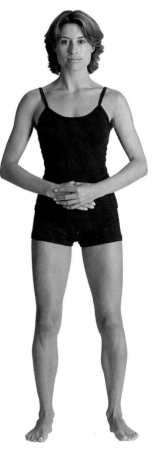

1 *Stand in the basic posture. Place your hands in front of your lower abdomen with your palms facing toward each other. Imagine that your hands are encircling a ball of energy that emanates from your lower dantien. Stay in this position for two minutes.*

2 *Move your hands slowly and sensitively a shoulders' width apart. Imagine as you do so that a ball of energy is expanding between your hands, gently pushing them out. Remain in this position for one minute, sensing the energy between your hands.*

3 *Imagine the ball of energy contracting, pulling your hands toward each other as it becomes more concentrated.*
Repeat this exercise several times, until you are aware of the change of sensation in your hands as they move apart and together. You may also feel a sensation within your abdomen, as if the energy is expanding and contracting in rhythm with your hands.

4 *Contract the ball of energy until it fits inside your abdomen. Tuck one hand inside the other, and touch your abdomen. As the energy contracts further, imagine it becoming a tiny bright light in the lower dantien. Release and shake your hands.*

STRENGTHENING THE FLOW OF ENERGY

One of the most important reasons for Qigong practice is to keep the energy flowing freely throughout your body. This graceful and flowing exercise is designed to make you feel energized, harmonized, and "clear." In general, the more you practice the greater the effect, but common sense should prevail. If you have serious physical limitations, for example, you should be guided by your instincts. If on the other hand you wish to stop the exercise from a sense of lethargy, it is worth continuing until the quality of the exercise changes and you can happily continue.

Your hands do not touch your body, but with practice you should increasingly be able to feel the connection between the two, and to sense the energy flowing over and through you. The exercise may be done slowly and meditatively or at a faster pace, placing greater emphasis on the movement.

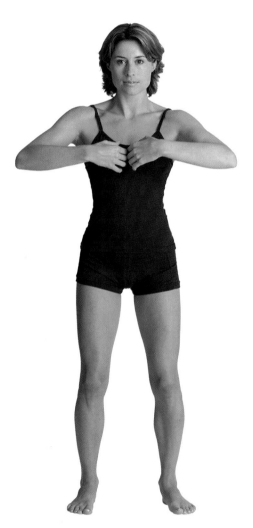

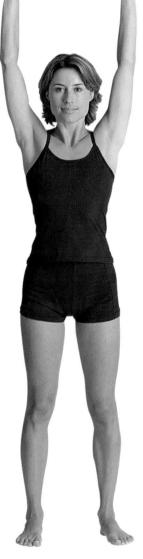

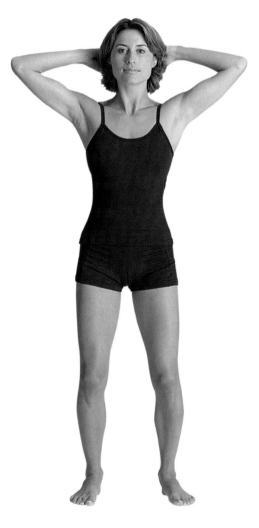

1 *Stand in the basic posture (see page 24). Raise your hands so that they face your lower abdomen, with your fingers slightly curled and pointing downward. Draw your hands up your body until they reach the breast, and point your fingers inward.*

2 *Keeping your shoulders relaxed, stretch your arms out on both sides. Then, with your palms facing forward, raise your arms above your head. Stretch as far as you can upward, allowing your heels to leave the ground if you wish.*

3 *Bring your hands down behind your head, cradling the area around your skull with your palms. Make sure that you follow the contours of your body with your hands, feeling the energy connection between both surfaces.*

6 Bring your hands over your hip joints and down the outside of your legs to the ground. Sweep around in front of your feet, and bring your hands back up the inside of your legs to your lower abdomen.
   Repeat 20 times stages 1 to 6, gradually increasing the number of times to 100.

CONCLUSION

The last time you bring your hands behind your head, continue to lower them, palms down, in front of your body. Imagine you are pushing the energy down your body and legs. Do not bend over. When your arms are almost straight hold the position (palms down) for about three minutes. Feel as if your hands are resting on your feet.
   Now, swing your arms across the front of your body, as if you are cutting the bonds between your hands and feet. Repeat nine times. Finish by shaking your hands, feet, and whole body.

4 Continue with your hands down the back of your neck and over your shoulders. Turn your hands and carry on down your chest with your palms facing inward and your fingers pointed toward your spine. Descend to your lower rib cage.

5 Take your hands around to your back and place them each side of your spine, just above the waist, behind the lower ribs. Your palms will be over the kidney area.

OVERCOMING BLOCKAGES IN THE MERIDIANS

Most of us constantly have blockages in our meridian network, the energy system that flows through our bodies (see pages 18–19). Although we are normally unaware of these blockages, sometimes they cause us pain or distress. We might then visit an Acupuncturist, who can release the block using a needle (see page 103).

This exercise is designed to relieve blockages in the meridians without needles, by sending the energy through the channels. It works systematically through the body, but if you have a specific blockage or problem you may need to concentrate more time and effort in one area. Generally, you should work on each area or limb until you feel a change in the quality of energy flowing through your body. Follow this exercise in the order suggested. Then choose those areas that are most in need of attention and repeat the appropriate stages.

1 *Give your body a good shake and shrug your shoulders to relax. Gently tap all over your head with your fingertips and then smooth it with your palms.*

Gently slap your left shoulder. Smooth down the outside of your left arm to your little finger ten times, to improve the flow of energy in your small intestine and heart meridians. Then repeat on your right shoulder and arm ten times.

2 *Gently tap the upper part of your chest, either side of your breastbone, with your fingertips. This will help to clear stagnation in the chest and to strengthen the lungs and respiratory system.*

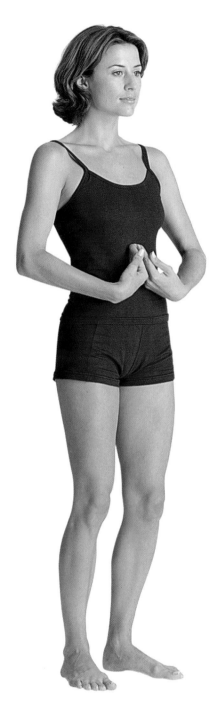

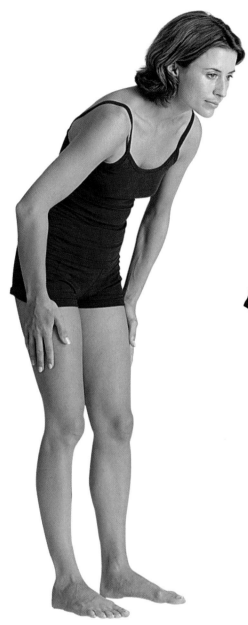

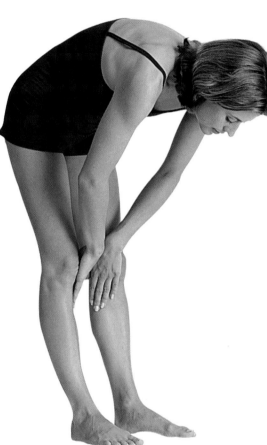

3 *Smooth down your body's midline with your fingertips facing toward your spine. This movement is working on the central channel, which helps to balance the Yin and Yang energies in the body (see pages 20–21). Repeat stages 2 and 3 another ten times.*

4 *Gently slap your hip joints, then smooth down the outside of your legs to the ground (bend your knees if necessary) and over your feet. This helps to clear blockages in the gall bladder and bladder meridians, which have been associated with conditions such as lower back pain, sciatica, period pain, and headaches. Be careful not to press the hips too hard or you may inflame the sciatic nerve.*

5 *Straighten up, bringing your hands up on the inside of your legs. Smooth up and down your legs another ten times.*
Stand in the basic posture for a few minutes, sensing the tingling in your body. Now comb down your arms, from your shoulder to just past your fingertips, about 4 inches (10 cm) from your skin. Comb one arm, then the other, ten times. Shake your arms and the rest of your body.

ACHIEVING AND MAINTAINING BALANCE

Balance is of the greatest importance when practicing Qigong. The ways in which we hold ourselves, walk and stand, bend and stretch should all be in balance. Some people spend years unconsciously holding one shoulder higher than the other or putting all their weight on one leg when they are standing still. This inevitably has a knock-on effect on their skeleton and muscle development. By being more aware of our bodies, we can become more in control and centered.

This exercise concentrates on balancing one side of the body with the other, so that gradually we become accustomed to a more symmetrical posture. The energy can flow equally on both sides and we can have greater flexibility. When you are stretching out sideways, feel as if your body is in two halves and imagine there is space down the middle: this is the "central channel." Once the central channel is opened, it affects the energy flow through the body.

Follow this exercise sensitively, experiencing the connection of energy between your hands and your body. As you stretch out, feel the energy flow along your arms and imagine your whole body is being pleasantly stretched apart and opened up.

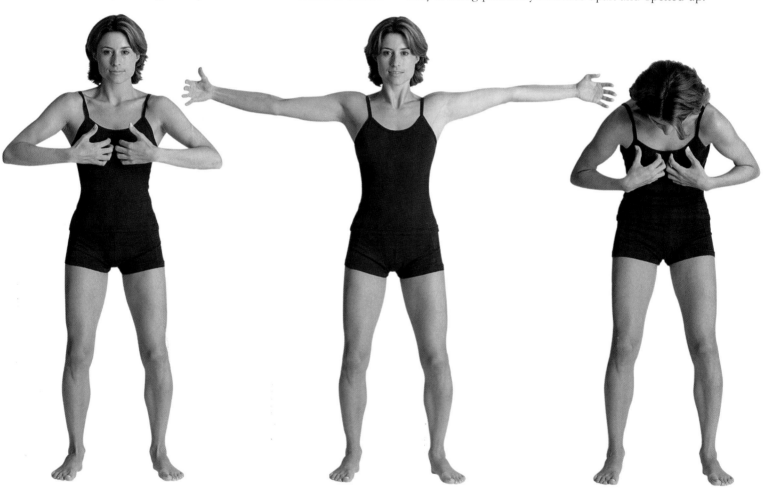

1 Stand with your feet parallel and a shoulders' width apart. Unlock your knees and tip your pelvis slightly forward. Keep your head erect. Curl your fingers and point them into your body, either side of your breastbone.

2 Without moving your feet, fully extend your arms both sides of your body, as if you are unfolding a scroll. Imagine that there is an energy-filled space between the two halves of your body. Remember to keep your shoulders relaxed.

3 Fold your arms in again, pointing your fingers toward your spine, and bend your head forward. Feel the stretch in your shoulders. Extend your arms again as in stage 2. Repeat 15 times, ending with the starting position (stage 1).

ROTATING A BALL OF ENERGY INSIDE YOUR ABDOMEN

This exercise uses the energy between your palms to help accumulate and conserve the Qi in your lower dantien (see page 25), the energy center in your abdomen. By rotating a ball of energy in front of your abdomen, you will be able to increase the amount of Qi in your body. This exercise is therefore extremely beneficial when you are feeling tired, run down, or generally lacking in energy. It is important to focus on your lower dantien, feeling the energy accumulate, when performing this exercise.

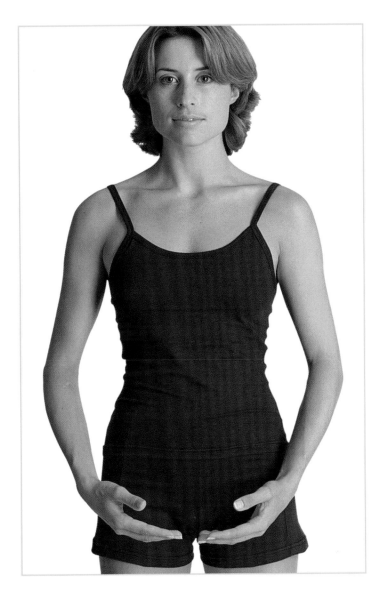

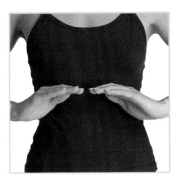

2 *Breathing naturally in through your nose and out through your mouth, slowly rotate your hands up and around the ball. Imagine that you are penetrating down inside your body.*

3 *Keep rotating your hands until they are resting on top of the ball, just below your ribs. Then bring your hands, thumbs first, around the back of the ball. Feel as if you are creating space in your body.*

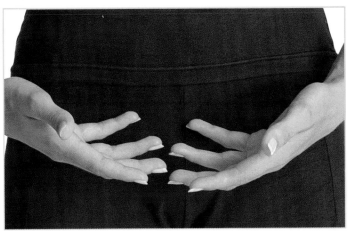

1 *Stand in the basic posture (see page 24). Hold your hands in front of your pelvic area with your palms facing upward and your fingers almost touching. Sense the connection between your hands and the energy within your lower dantien. Remain in this position for two minutes, imagining the energy is growing and filling out into a ball of energy within your hands.*

4 *As your hands reach the lowest level, in front of your pelvic area, twist them so they are beneath the energy ball. Rotate the ball another 35 times. Finally, with your hands in position 1, imagine the ball of energy contracting into a tiny spark of light within the lower dantien. Shake your hands when you have finished this exercise.*

ENERGY IN THE JAPANESE TRADITION

Japanese ideas of energy have been influenced by Daoist and other practices from China. However, they are also closely linked to the religious traditions of Shintoism and Buddhism in Japan itself. The whole focus is on working with energy to facilitate physical, mental, and spiritual development.

In Japan there is also an emphasis on harmony and balance, both within the individual and between the individual and the environment. Japan's most ancient religion Shinto, meaning "the way of the gods," teaches that gods or *kami* may reside in all things, including people, animals, trees, rocks, and mountains. As a result, there is a great respect for nature in Japan. An understanding of how it operates—both universally in the macrocosm and within the individual in the microcosm—has resulted from these beliefs.

As in Chinese ideas of energy, the ultimate energy is conceived of as the oneness of the universe. This cosmic energy is differentiated by the relative influence of Yin and Yang, two opposing yet complementary forces (see page 20). Further variation occurs due to the influence of the five basic elements—water, wood, fire, earth, and metal—that constitute all natural phenomena. In the physical body the diversity of this energy manifests itself as the different internal organs, the meridian system of energetic channels, and the energetic centers known in the Indian system as the chakras (see page 44).

The mysteries of the universe, including the concepts of convergent opposites (Yin-Yang), are illustrated in Japanese Zen gardens, which are designed as meditative tools. By deliberating on an area of gravel that is raked to suggest water, or a barren landscape that is punctuated

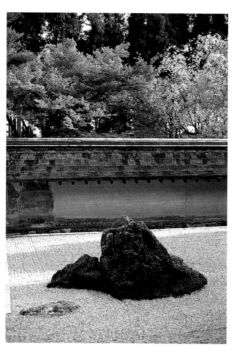

Part of the famous Zen rock garden at the 15th-century Ryoan-ji temple in Kyoto in Japan.

by a number of rocks, a meditating Zen Buddhist may suddenly come to understand the connection between matter and emptiness, permanence and impermanence, the relative and the absolute.

The Japanese word for the energy coursing through the body's meridians is Ki (pronounced "kee," the equivalent to the Chinese Qi). It can be translated as "vital force," the intangible, essential energy that pervades all living things. In Japanese, Ki provides the root for many words. "Gen-ki," which means good, flowing Ki or "health"; "byo-ki," meaning blocked or damaged Ki or "disease"; and "ten-ki," meaning heavenly Ki or "weather," all illustrate the wide application of this concept.

In traditional Japanese medicine the Ki, or vital spirit, is said to reside in the abdomen or *hara*. More specifically, the energy is centered at a point (the tanden) about three fingers' width below the navel, which corresponds to the Chinese lower dantien (see page 25). It is at the *hara* that all the vital processes of the body's support systems are initiated and where each of the meridians is represented. It is considered vital to maintain energy in the *hara* and to operate from the *hara* when executing movements. For this reason the *hara* is emphasized in all Japanese martial arts.

The various forms of self-regulatory exercise systems (such as Do-in), the traditional healing and medical techniques (including Shiatsu) and martial arts (including Kendo, Aikido, and Judo) that exist within Japan are all based on the concept of promoting the free-flow of Ki and improving its circulation in the body. It is firmly held that this will strengthen both mind and body, prevent disease, and help develop individual potential.

ENERGY AND THE MARTIAL ARTS

There are two broad types of martial arts: those that are armed and those that are unarmed. Among the former are Kyudo (archery) and Kendo (fencing); the latter group uses the body itself as a means of defence or attack.

Traditionally, a Japanese warrior's training would include archery, swordsmanship, and unarmed combat. They also had to be able to swim in armor. Some of the best warriors were Ninjas, who were skilled in Ninjutsu. This martial art, practiced by military spies in feudal Japan, was characterized by the adepts' stealthy movements and camouflage.

Today, the modern derivatives of the unarmed forms of combat, such as Judo, Sumo, and Karate, have become popular throughout the world, as have non-aggressive forms of self-defence, such as Aikido and Hapkido.

In Japan the martial arts are practiced not only as a method of self-defence, but also as a means of energy-building and spiritual development. This is due in part to the influence of both Zen Buddhism and Daoism, and their strong emphasis on the mental and spiritual state of the practitioner. By suspending the constant questioning and rationalizing functions of the mind, a state of higher consciousness can be entered, enabling the mind and body to work together in a harmony of intent and action.

Many adherents to Zen Buddhism and Daoism practice the martial arts as part of their philosophical and spiritual training. Conversely, many practitioners of the martial arts become followers of these philosophies.

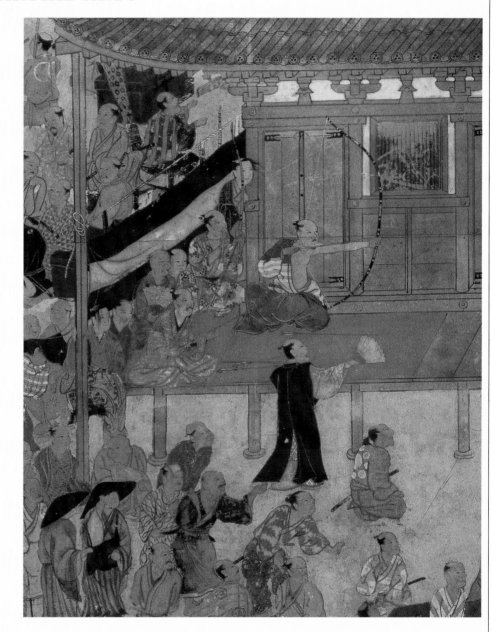

Archers in Japan learned to be at one with their bows and yet to be detached from the outcome of their shot. This state of "no-thought," known as mushin, *was achieved through the inner balance of the mind and the outer mastery of the body.*

This painting, which dates from the Momoyama period (1574–1600), depicts samurai, monks, and townspeople at an archery contest.

DO-IN

The Japanese term Do-in means "self-regulation and adjustment," and it relates to a system of ancient exercises for harmonious physical, mental, and spiritual development. The system originated in China, but was further developed in Japan by linking it with local esoteric and religious practices.

The uniqueness of the exercises is that they are performed by an individual on him- or herself, without the need for other people or special equipment, and they are intuitive and far-reaching in their effects. The aim of the exercises is to develop not only your physical health but also your mental and spiritual abilities. The ultimate aim of Do-in is to improve society and the world.

The exercises can be practiced any time and anywhere, so they can easily be built into your daily routine. Many of them are stationary and introspective, designed to develop self-awareness and mental faculties. Others involve moving sequences, such as walking and ritual dances, which should be performed daily to stimulate Ki circulation and enhance personal vitality.

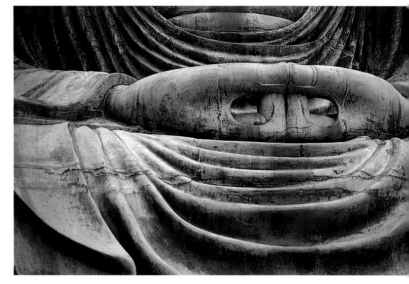

A detail from the bronze statue known as Daibitsu or the "Great Buddha" at Kamakura in Japan. Cast in 1252, it is 37 ft (11 m) high, and shows the Buddha Amida, who governs the Pure Land, a Buddhist paradise.

TEN-DAI BUDDHISM

Ten-dai Buddhism was adapted and brought to Japan from China during the 8th century by a Buddhist monk known as Saicho. The first Ten-dai temple was erected on Mount Hiei, to the east of Kyoto. Mount Hiei is also important to the followers of the Shinto religion, who believe that gods are manifest in the natural world, as it is said to be guarded by the Shinto spirit "The King of the Mountain."

From Mount Hiei, Saicho taught his monks three main beliefs. Firstly, that everybody had the ability to reach Buddhahood. This was a breakthrough for Japanese Buddhism, which had become centered on the wealthy, well-educated minority. Secondly, Saicho insisted that monks spend 12 years in the monastery practicing concentration and insight. This was an unusually harsh regime that emphasized the need for inner harmony. Saicho's third belief was that his monks had a duty to encourage loyalty and national pride in those whom they taught.

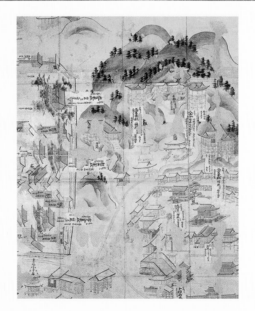

An 18th-century map from the Edo period showing Ten-dai Buddhist shrines and temples on Mount Hiei.

HEAVENLY FOUNDATION (TEN-DAI)

This exercise helps to unite Heaven and Earth energies in the body. Daily practice of Ten-dai helps to develop confidence, will, and calm faith. By touching your index fingers with your thumbs you are symbolizing the union of the individual "I" (the index finger) with the universal "One" (the thumb). The straight spine enables energy to flow freely from the vital energy centers in the head to nourish the tanden and energy center in the lower abdomen. Known as the lower dantien in the Chinese system, the tanden is said to be the seat of vitality in the body; it corresponds to the second chakra (see page 45). Its approximate location is three fingers' width below the navel.

If you find kneeling in this position for a long time uncomfortable, place a small rolled blanket or towel under your thighs. Alternatively, meditate sitting upright on a chair with your knees slightly apart and your feet placed flat on the floor.

Kneel on a soft surface with your knees a fist's width apart, your big toes overlapping, and your buttocks placed in between your heels (this aids circulation and so prevents numbness). Rest your palms on your upper thighs, with your hands pointing slightly inward and your thumbs tucked in to lightly touch your index fingers. Keep your spine straight throughout this exercise.

Gently close your eyes and relax. Focus your concentration inward to the tanden energy field in the middle of the lower abdomen.

Breathe in deeply through your nose and draw the breath down into the lower abdomen, allowing it to expand slightly. Hold for one or two seconds. Contract the abdomen and exhale through the nose. Repeat this slow, rhythmical breathing for several minutes. As you breathe in, concentrate on drawing energy in from above and sending it down to the lower abdomen. As you hold the breath and then exhale, focus your concentration downward, feeling your link with the Earth.

Open your eyes and stretch your arms above your head. Now relax them by your sides and stretch out your legs.

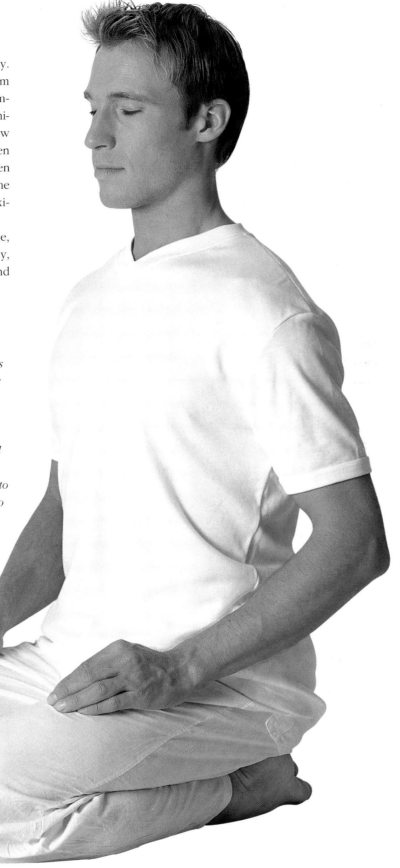

SHIATSU

Shiatsu, meaning "finger pressure," is a form of therapeutic massage and manipulation that has been developed in Japan over the last 100 years. It involves the application of pressure to the meridian lines and acupoints of the body in order to regulate the flow of Ki. Many parts of the body—including the thumbs, fingertips, palms, elbows, knees, and even feet—may be used to apply the pressure.

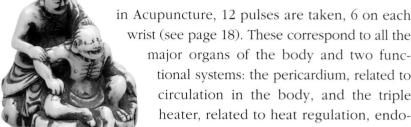

The benefits of massage have long been known in Japan, as demonstrated by this 18th- or 19th-century netsuke.

In Japan, Shiatsu is an accepted medical therapy used to prevent and treat disease. Traditionally, many practitioners were blind and had a highly developed sense of touch, but today most are sighted. Some have incorporated elements of Western massage and physiotherapy into their Shiatsu practice, so it is therefore a continually evolving form of therapy.

In Shiatsu, diagnosis is made by feeling for the flow of Ki energy at the site of acupoints, along the meridian lines, in the area of the abdomen, and at the pulses. As in Acupuncture, 12 pulses are taken, 6 on each wrist (see page 18). These correspond to all the major organs of the body and two functional systems: the pericardium, related to circulation in the body, and the triple heater, related to heat regulation, endocrine, and sexual function within the body.

Steady, continuous pressure applied to the acupoints, meridian lines, or abdomen also forms the basis of treatment, which opens acupoints, unblocks channels, and stimulates vital organ function. Changes can also be made directly to the body's nervous and immune systems.

Some Shiatsu may be performed on oneself, but most needs to be carried out by another. Qualified practitioners have studied for at least a year and many have also trained in Acupuncture or other forms of massage. However, some simple techniques can be learned easily by lay people and have enormous health benefits.

ACUPOINTS ON THE FINGERTIPS

Each fingertip is the start or end point of a major meridian, which crosses the fingers and hands and runs along the arms. The small intestine meridian not only deals with digestion but is also said to discriminate between what is and is not needed by the body. The heart meridian sends nourishment in the form of blood and Ki throughout the body. The triple heater, which ensures the proper movement of Ki and fluids in the body, is not recognized in Western medicine. The pericardium, also known as the heart protector, covers the heart, shielding it from psychological disturbances. The large intestine meridian is connected with elimination and contraction, and the lung meridian governs the reception and regulation of of Ki from the air.

This diagram shows the acupoints of the six meridians that run through the hands. The left hand is shown here, but the points on the right hand form a mirror image, so that there is also a lung meridian acupoint on the thumb of the right hand.

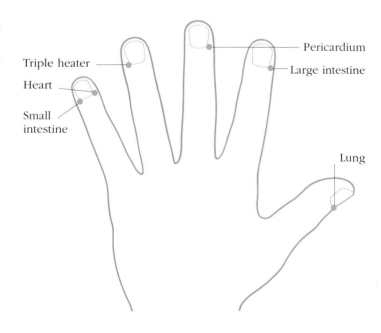

SHIATSU FINGER MASSAGE

Our fingers are highly sensitive and, if massaged, can help to relieve tension or stress throughout our bodies. By applying Shiatsu along each of the fingers and stimulating the acupoints in the fingertips, the flow of Ki in their corresponding meridians is improved. This finger massage should be done sitting comfortably, with your shoulders and neck relaxed so that you can breathe freely. Your elbows should be raised so that your forearms form a straight line across your chest.

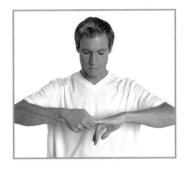 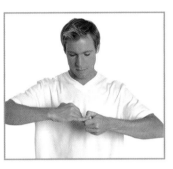

1 *With your left palm face down, grasp the base of your left little finger between the thumb (flat on top of finger) and index finger (bent beneath finger) of your right hand. Squeeze along the little finger to the tip, while exerting an opposing force by pulling away slightly with the left arm.*

2 *At the fingertip carry on supporting with your index finger and apply pressure to the nail bed using the thumb.
Repeat the procedure for each of the fingers in turn, moving from the little finger to the thumb, and then do the same for the opposite hand, starting with the little finger.*

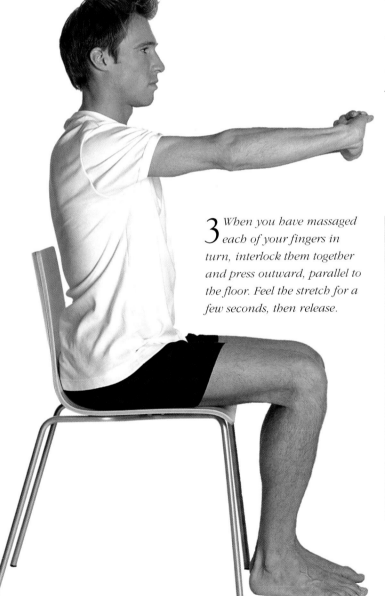

3 *When you have massaged each of your fingers in turn, interlock them together and press outward, parallel to the floor. Feel the stretch for a few seconds, then release.*

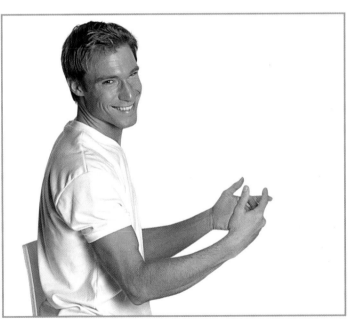

4 *Shake your wrists freely with the fingers loose. Now rest your hands on your lap, close your eyes, and focus on the pleasant tingling sensation in your fingers, hands, and arms. You should feel an increase of heat and energy in these areas.*

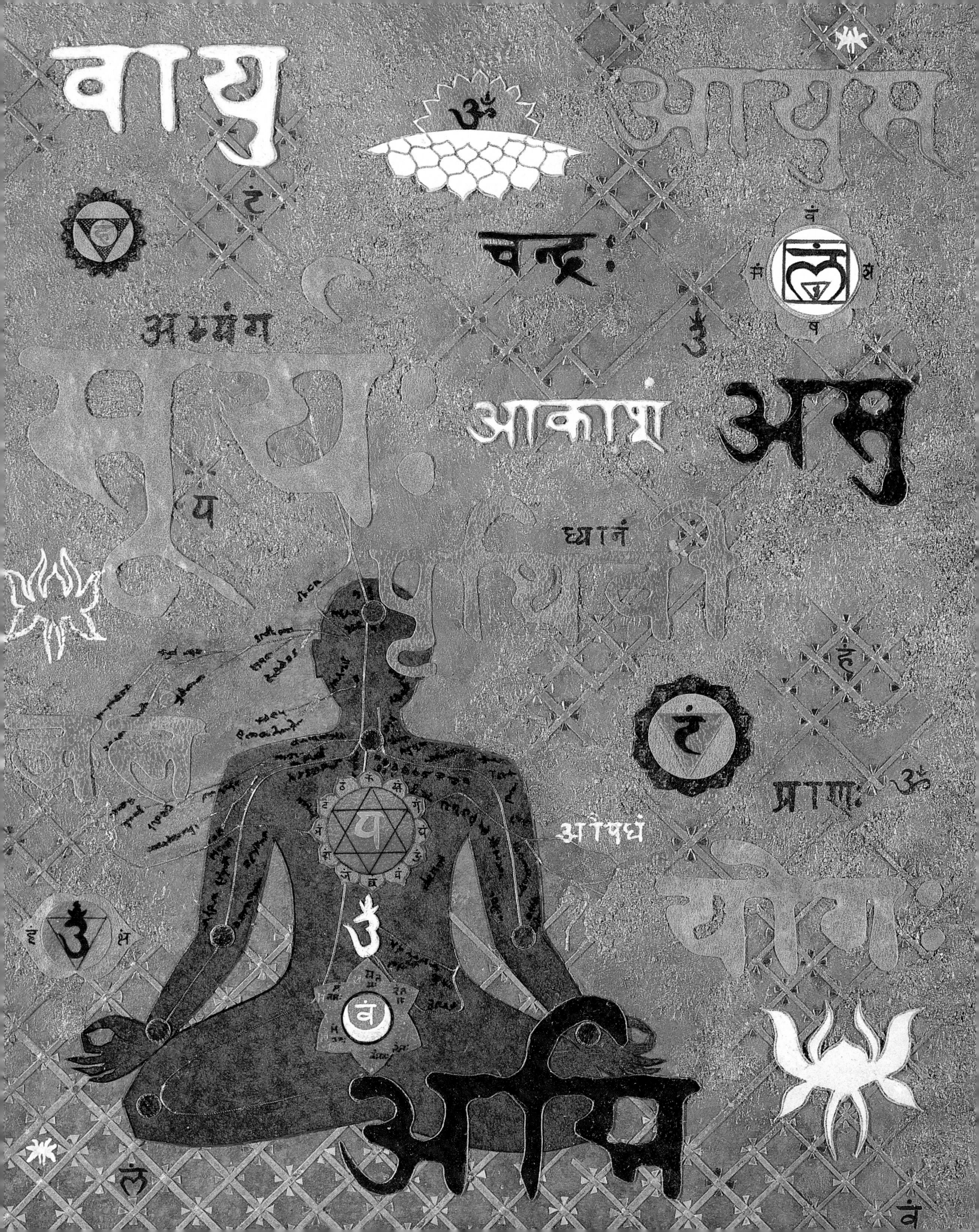

वायु
चन्द्रः
आकाशं
प्राणः
अग्नि

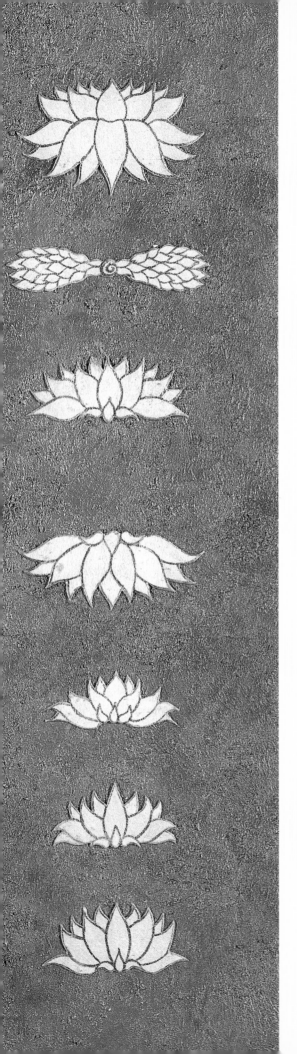

INDIAN IDEAS OF ENERGY

In the Indian tradition, the health of the body is governed by the flow of Prana, or "vital energy," through channels known as *nadis*. If Prana is flowing effectively, then the body will remain healthy. However, if it is hindered or blocked, then disease will eventually result.

Asanas (postures), *pranayama* (breathing exercises), and *dhyana* (meditation practices) are steps used in Hatha Yoga to remove the energy blockages in the body and to control and stimulate the flow of Prana. By practicing all three steps it is possible for an adept to make their body into a perfect instrument.

Hindus believe that by controlling the body and calming the mind it is possible to see the spirit or true self. When this is achieved, release from the bondage of birth, death, and the illusions of everyday life is possible.

INDIAN CONCEPTS OF ENERGY

The Hindu tradition has incorporated and formalized many of the ancient Vedic beliefs about energy and the universe. Modern Hindus have evolved a complete system of personal development that encompasses the energy of the body, mind, and spirit. The system is based on the belief that the universe is a manifestation of one absolute reality, or consciousness, known as Brahman. Uncreated, limitless, all-embracing, and eternal, Brahman underlies the universe and everything in it, including the *atman* or soul of each individual. Hindus believe that if we recognize our true nature—that "I [the *atman*] am that consciousness [Brahman]"—then we will be freed from the illusory world of time, space, and causation, and become reunited with the Absolute (Brahman). Because we are all part of this consciousness, we can all train ourselves to access its infinite energy.

The fundamental principles of this system had begun to form by around 3,000 B.C.E. and were referred to in the *Vedas*, the sacred texts introduced to the Indus Valley by the Aryans. They were expanded in the *Upanishads*, a collection of texts that date from the 9th to the 5th centuries B.C.E., which recommended meditation, Yoga, and renunciation as paths to unite the individual soul with the Absolute. The 6th century B.C.E. also saw the appearance of two renowned epic Indian poems: the *Ramayana* and the *Mahabharata*. The latter incorporates the *Bhagavad Gita*, which synthesizes all the disciplines of Yoga, including Karma Yoga, Jnana Yoga, Bhakti Yoga, and Raja Yoga. This final path, sometimes translated as "Royal Yoga," is the form best known in the West today. It was first elaborated in the *Yoga Sutras* attributed to the sage Patanjali. Among the "eight limbs" of Raja Yoga (steps to purify the body and mind) are *asanas* (postures) and *pranayama* (breathing exercises). Both of these elements, emphasized in the subdivision known as Hatha Yoga, help to channel the body's vital energy, or Prana.

Prana is the life force that flows through all things, keeping them alive and well nourished. One of the most important ways that we take Prana into our own bodies is

THE ENERGY OF THE SUN

From earliest times, the Sun has been worshipped by men and women as the source of all life, light, and warmth on this planet. It has usually been seen as male and associated with positive, active qualities. For Hindus, the Sun is a symbol of humankind's higher self; the *Upanishads* speak of the souls of the knowing ascending after death to the Sun. The ancient practice of worshipping the Sun god Surya has been continued in the form of the Yoga exercise Salute to the Sun or *Surya namaskar* (see pages 52–3). When performing this graceful sequence of 12 variations adepts thank the Sun for its many benedictions and ask for their energy and strength to be increased. Each of the variations is associated with a sign of the Zodiac, further emphasizing the sequence's relationship with the heavens. Ideally, the sequence should be practiced 12 times every morning at dawn, in order that the energy of the rising Sun may be harnessed. Each round should be accompanied by the chanting of a different mantra praising the life-giving qualities of the Sun.

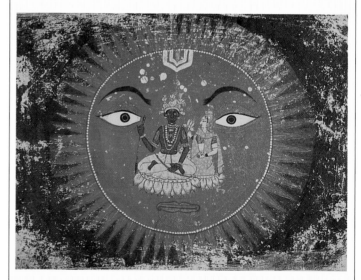

This 18th-century miniature painting, known as The Heart of Surya, *depicts the Vedic Sun god. To the ancient inhabitants of the Indian subcontinent, Surya was a powerful symbol of universal energy and provision.*

through breathing. Although some Prana is carried in our physical bodies, most flows through our subtle or astral bodies. As with meridian theory (see pages 18–19), good health depends on preserving the flow and balance of energy in the body and ill health results from a blockage in its flow. If the blockage is removed, then the body will return to a state of good health. Therefore, in the Indian traditions of Yoga and Ayurveda (see pages 118–21), emphasis is placed on living in harmony with nature and maintaining a good flow of Prana in order to prevent disease. Adepts learn five principles that lead to physical, mental, and spiritual health: proper exercise, proper breathing, proper relaxation, proper diet, and positive thinking and meditation.

MANTRAS

Mantras are sacred words, sounds, or symbols that have been used since ancient times to purify the mind. The Sanskrit word "mantra" is made up of two elements: "man" from *manana*, which means "thinking," and "tra" from *trana* or liberation. So mantras are sounds or words that free the mind. Every sound or word has a consciousness, energy, and vibration, which can be either beneficial or harmful. Here we are concerned with beneficial mantras.

The act of repeating a mantra is known as *japa*. If you perform *japa* constantly and devotedly, the meaning of the mantra starts to permeate your whole being. For example, if you devotedly repeat the word "peace" or the phrase "I am relaxed," and let the meaning of these words be absorbed into your body and mind, you will soon feel peaceful and relaxed. Similarly, when you repeat a holy mantra, such as OM, it gradually leads to the indwelling spirit of the word. The meaning of the mantra starts to become part of you, provoking a change within you, which may lead to a spiritual awakening. As you think, so you become.

Mantras can be repeated out loud, in a whisper, or silently. Traditionally, a rosary (*mala*) is used to record the number of times a mantra is repeated, but you may also keep count on your fingers or write the mantra down as you recite it.

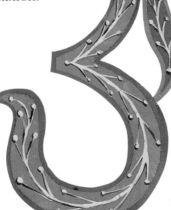

The stylized pictograph used to represent OM, the most sacred of sounds, is the most revered symbol in the Hindu world.

The relationship between the body, mind, and spirit is central to adepts of Hatha Yoga, who believe that the spirit can be liberated by controlling the body and mind. Hindu scriptures provide the analogy of a chariot to explain the order of the spirit, mind, and body. The five horses pulling the chariot are like the body's five senses. The chariot is the body and the mind is represented by the reins that are controlling the horses. The charioteer, the real controller, is the spirit. Using *asanas* and *pranayama* Yoga adepts are able to control the flow of Prana through their bodies. Then, through meditation they can calm their minds, enabling them to see things in their true perspective.

Mantras fall into three main categories: Saguna mantras, Nirguna mantras, and Bija mantras. Saguna mantras invoke a form, usually that of a deity, such as Krishna, Rama, or Sarasvati. Nirguna mantras are abstract and usually identify the reciter with different aspects of the Absolute. One example is SO HAM. As SO means "that Absolute" and HAM means "me," SO HAM can be translated as "I am the Absolute itself." Bija or "seed" mantras are various aspects of the supreme mantra OM. They are derived from the 50 primeval sounds of the Sanskrit language. Examples of Bija mantras include the individual seed sounds of the chakras (see page 45). It is said that each element of the universe has its own corresponding seed sound.

OM is the root mantra, the sound that represents cosmic consciousness, the Absolute. OM is also known as Pranava, or Life Force, because it pervades everything. Just as white is the synthesis of all the colors of the light spectrum, so OM is regarded as the synthesis of all the cosmic vibrations. It pervades every sound and every mantra. The OM sound is divided into three syllables: A-U-M. "A" is the guttural sound that comes out of the mouth when it is first opened. It represents the awake state. "U" represents the middle range, the dream state. "M" is the last sound formed as the lips are closed, and is symbolic of the sleeping state.

ENERGY, BREATHING, AND MEDITATION

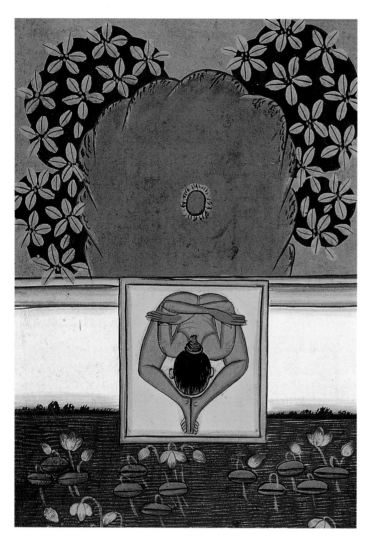

An illustration from an 18th-century Hatha Yoga textbook showing a Hindu ascetic performing an asana, *or posture, recommended for meditation.*

Breathing is an instinctive and involuntary process, and yet many of us do not realize the physical and mental benefits to be gained from breathing properly. By using a greater surface area of our lungs when we breathe, we increase the amount of oxygen absorbed into our bodies. Oxygen is an essential ingredient in the metabolism of each of the body's cells, and increasing the amount absorbed can improve our metabolic rate; in the brain this can lead to greater powers of concentration.

Yogis believe that there is another reason to breathe properly: to control the amount of Prana (vital energy) flowing through the body. As the mind also uses Prana to function, you can control the mind by controlling the flow of Prana in the body. Yogis perform *pranayama* (breathing exercises) to strengthen the body, clear the mind, and maintain inner harmony, thus preventing illness. When performing *pranayama*, Yogis both inhale and exhale solely through their noses. This is because the Ida and Pingala *nadis*, two of the main channels that carry Prana, flow through the nostrils. By choosing to breathe through a particular nostril, and stopping the other nostril with a finger, Yogis are able to determine into which channel the Prana is absorbed, and so to balance their bodies' energy by regulating their breathing.

There is a direct correlation between a person's state of mind and his or her respiratory pattern. If someone is agitated then the breathing will be shallow, uneven, and fast. But if his or her outlook is calm and serene, the pattern of breathing is likely to be deep, regular, and quiet. By focusing attention on our breathing, we can gradually slow it down, making it more regular and deeper. This has the effect of calming the mind. When the mind becomes still we are able to see our true spirit and are said to be in a meditative state.

Meditation (*dhyana*) is thus the practice of relaxing the body and quieting the mind in order to see the true self as part of the Absolute. In physical terms it has been proved to reduce the heart rate, which in turn reduces recognizable levels of stress.

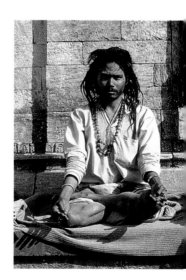

A Hindu fakir meditates in the lotus position. His pose provides a firm base to contain the flow of Prana. His thumbs and index fingers are joined in the Chin mudra, *forming an "O" that signifies the unity of all things.*

ENERGY CHANNELS

Prana, or vital energy, is carried around the subtle body in channels known as *nadis*. Because illness is believed to result from the *nadis* being blocked, Hindus have developed Yoga *asanas* (postures) and *pranayama* (breathing exercises) to purify and strengthen the channels. There are 72,000 *nadis* in the body, the most important of which is the Sushumna, whose equivalent in the physical body is the spinal cord.

Flanking the Sushumna are the Ida and Pingala *nadis*, which can be accessed through the nostrils. Normally, these two *nadis* carry most of the body's Prana, and it is only during meditation that the body's Kundalini energy is aroused and directed into the Sushumna (see page 44). The Ida *nadi* is the left nostril channel and is related to the cooling Moon energy. It controls the left side of the body and the right side of the brain, which is calming, intuitive, and emotional. The right nostril channel is the Pingala *nadi*, which is related to the warming Sun energy. It controls the right side of the body and the left side of the brain, which is logical and rational. Breathing through just one nostril will alter the balance of energy in the body.

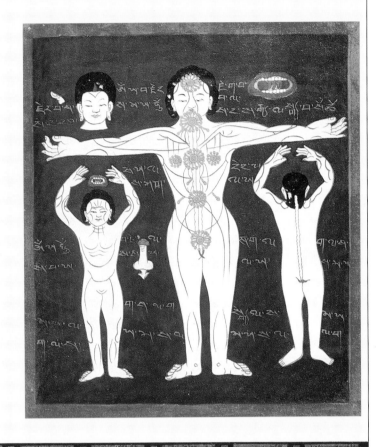

A Nepalese painting showing the body's channels and centers of breath control. Balancing the energy flow in these channels is believed to lead to health, longevity, and spiritual enlightenment.

According to Patanjali, who is regarded as the Father of Yoga, the first step to controlling the mind is to concentrate on one thing to the exclusion of everything else. Concentration (*dharana*) enables a person to discard the influence of his or her senses and intuitively to penetrate and examine the object of study. This object will then begin to magnify and take the meditator to deeper levels of consciousness. Practical advice on Yogic meditation is given on pages 134–5.

Positive thinking is another important strand of Yoga. If an individual persistently thinks positively, then he or she will gain wisdom and inner peace. To do this he or she must first let go of any conscious thoughts, feelings, and actions, and learn to accept that the only true reality is the Absolute.

By discovering the truth that there is only one reality, and feeling the connection between the individual and the Absolute, negative emotions (such as apprehension, grief, and hate) will vanish. It is the aim of all those who practice Yoga to achieve this state of release. If, through meditation and positive thinking, they succeed in purifying the mind, then the Absolute will act through the individual. This, however, takes a great deal of discipline and selflessness. In the *Bhagavad Gita* ("Song of the Blessed One"), from the epic poem the *Mahabharata*, the Lord Krishna states that the "Mind, although very difficult to control by *abhyasa* (practice) and *vairagya* (dispassion), can be controlled." Yet in order to control the mind, we have first to develop a strong will. The greatest obstacle in our way is usually our pursuit of pleasure.

THE SUBTLE BODY AND ITS CHAKRAS

In addition to the physical body, Hindus teach that men and women possess both a subtle or astral body and a causal body. The subtle body interpenetrates and extends just beyond the physical body. It is made up of a network of *nadis* (channels, see page 43) through which Prana (vital energy) flows, and which house the mind and intellect. The subtle and physical bodies are connected by a thread, which is severed when the physical bodies dies. The causal body is linked to the other two bodies. It contains the seeds of the soul and remains with the subtle body after death.

The chakras are seven centers of energy in the subtle body that correspond to nerve centers in the physical body. They are located along the Sushumna *nadi*, the central energy channel in the subtle body, which ascends

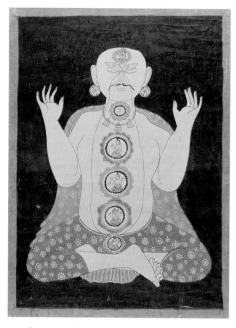

In this Nepalese painting the seven chakras are depicted along the midline of the body. Each has a sacred image at its center.

from the base chakra or Muladhara, to the crown chakra or Sahasrara. The chakras are the main receptors and distributors of Prana in the subtle body. Each is thought to vibrate at a particular frequency as it sends Prana around the body.

Each chakra has been associated with a particular type of consciousness. The lower two centers are associated with the animalistic qualities of humankind and govern stimuli such as eating, drinking, and sexual pleasure. The solar, heart, and throat chakras are responsible for feeding the emotions and those mental functions that together make up the personality. The brow and the crown chakras are related to intuition, integration, and enlightenment.

Recently, a link has been made between the chakras and the location and functioning of the major nerve

KUNDALINI

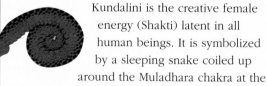

Kundalini is the creative female energy (Shakti) latent in all human beings. It is symbolized by a sleeping snake coiled up around the Muladhara chakra at the base of the central channel or Sushumna *nadi*.

Kundalini Yoga is an attempt to fuse the male and female creative forces within an individual. By using breathing techniques (*pranayama*, see page 42) and meditation (*dhyana*, see pages 134–5) an adept creates an inner heat that rouses the serpent power from its sleep. This energy then rises up the

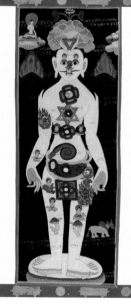

Sushumna, piercing each of the chakras in its path and absorbing their energy. The adept enters a higher state of consciousness as each chakra is passed. Eventually the serpent power reaches the crown chakra where Shiva (consciousness) resides. If the male and female energies of Shiva and Shakti fully unite, then the adept attains liberation from the illusions of everyday life.

An 18th-century painting in Nepalese style of a Cosmic Man. A snake is slowly uncoiling between the second and third chakras.

plexuses of the physical body. Each of the latter is related to one of the endocrine glands, which secrete hormones directly into the bloodstream. If the energy in a chakra is imbalanced, then it is thought to affect the corresponding gland, causing hormonal levels to fluctuate. This can alter a person's libido, heart rate, blood pressure, blood sugar, metabolism, growth and development, mood, and sleep pattern. Physical and emotional health are therefore only possible if all the chakras are functioning well.

Like the meridians (see pages 18–19), the chakras function together rather than in isolation. If one chakra malfunctions, it will cause an energy blockage that affects the other six. Hindus believe that physical and emotional imbalances should therefore be addressed immediately, in order to maintain a good flow of energy and so remain healthy. Three ways of regulating flow are *asanas* (postures), *pranayama* (breathing exercises), and meditation.

DEPICTING THE CHAKRAS

The seven chakras are positioned along the Sushumna, the central channel of the subtle body. Traditionally, each chakra is depicted as a lotus with a different number of petals, which is said to relate to the number of *nadis* that run through them. Symbols and seed mantras (see page 41) are associated with all but the crown chakra, which represents the Absolute and so is impossible to define. The five lower chakras have also been associated with the five elements. Various colors have been used by different schools of thought to describe the energy pattern of each chakra, but they can be linked to the colors of the light spectrum, as shown in the table below. Under this system the energy of the base chakra is red, a color usually associated with rawness, and the energy of the crown chakra is violet, a sign of spirituality.

Sahasrara (crown) chakra

Ajna (brow) chakra

Vishuddha (throat) chakra

Anahata (heart) chakra

Manipura (solar) chakra

Swadhishthana (navel) chakra

Muladhara (root) chakra

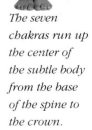

The seven chakras run up the center of the subtle body from the base of the spine to the crown.

NAME	Muladhara (Root center)	Swadhishthana (Navel center)	Manipura (Solar center)	Anahata (Heart center)	Vishuddha (Throat center)	Ajna (Brow center)	Sahasrara (Crown center)
LOCATION	Perineum	Sacrum/genitals	Solar plexus	Heart	Throat	Brow	Crown
SYMBOL	Square	Crescent moon	Triangle	Star of David	Inverted triangle	OM	–
LOTUS PETALS	4	6	10	12	16	2	1,000
ELEMENT	Earth	Water	Fire	Air	Ether	–	–
SEED SOUND	Lam	Vam	Ram	Yam	Ham	OM	–
COLOR	Red	Orange	Yellow	Green	Blue	Indigo	Violet

HATHA YOGA

Hatha Yoga is the school of Yoga best known in the West, and emphasizes the physical aspects of Yoga. Hatha is made up of two words: "Ha," meaning positive, and "Tha," meaning negative. Hatha Yoga is therefore a means of balancing the positive and negative energies in the body. It does this through *asanas* (postures), *pranayama* (breathing exercises), *mudras* (hand positions that channel the Prana in specific directions), *bandhas* (muscular "locks" that control the flow of Prana), and *kriyas* (internal cleansing practices).

Priority is given to effective breathing techniques and to the proper synchronization of each breath with each movement. When practicing Yoga you should breathe through your nostrils. Great emphasis is placed on exhalation because the more that you breathe out, the more stale air you are removing from your system.

Yoga's main aim is to nourish the body and mind rather than to burn energy in the form of calories. Ayurveda (see pages 118–21) and Hatha Yoga's overall approach to exercise is that it should be gentle and should not strain the body. After a session you should feel nourished and revitalized, not exhausted.

In Yoga, the word *asana* (posture) is used rather than exercise. This implies stillness. The aim is to get into a posture and then to relax into it and to become that posture. All Yogic postures form a circuit of energy. If an adept relaxes into the posture, then he or she can plug into the healing energy that is naturally available within us. Each posture also creates a certain state of mind.

If you are to make progress in Yoga, you have to want to improve and so should practice with devotion every day. The level of progress you are likely to make will depend on the intensity of your practice and devotion.

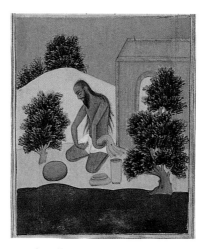

In this illustration from a Sanskrit book on Yoga, translated into Persian c.1800, an adept is depicted in a standard Yogic pose.

It is important that you build up your Yoga practice gradually; do not exceed your own physical limitations. Everybody is at a different stage in their physical and spiritual development, so there is no point in comparing your abilities with another's. Yoga can be practiced by anyone, regardless of age, sex, or state of fitness.

However, if you do have a medical disorder, it is important that you check with your doctor before attempting the *asanas*. The Yoga exercises given in this book are designed as an introduction to the discipline but cannot replace the benefits of learning from a qualified Yoga teacher.

The best times to practice Yoga are before breakfast, lunch, or dinner. It is particularly beneficial in the morning, when the body tends to be a bit stiff. Never practice with a full stomach; wait at least four hours after a heavy meal and two hours after a light one.

No special clothing or equipment is necessary to practice Yoga, but it is better to wear loose, comfortable clothing so that you can move without restrictions. It is preferable to wear cotton rather than synthetic fibers, so that your skin can breathe freely. For the same reason, do not wear any shoes or socks on your feet.

A Yoga session should start with a few minutes of relaxation in the Shavasana, also known as the Corpse Pose (see page 133). Then do a few gentle warming-up stretches to loosen up the body. Pay particular attention to the hip joints, shoulder sockets, neck, and ankles. Standing postures warm up the body effectively. An advanced variation should always be preceded by preliminary warming-up exercises. If you complete a well-designed sequence of Yoga *asanas* properly, you will have systematically stretched every part of your body and massaged your internal organs and glands.

STANDING UPRIGHT (SAMASTHITI)

This is the basic standing posture from which all the standing postures begin and to which they all return. It is instrumental in the alignment of the body. Slouching, round shoulders, sagging stomach, arched back, and tilted head are only a few examples of bad posture, all of which interfere with the body's health.

When in the posture, feel as if you are firmly rooted in nature; that you are balanced, integrated, and at one with the universe. Stand full of confidence, with firmness and poise. Feel as if your body is a perfect instrument, waiting to be played.

The more you breathe out, the more toxins you will remove from your respiratory system. Then, when you breathe in, you will be replacing the toxins with clean, fresh air.

Although you should concentrate on increasing the period of exhalation, it is important not to strain your respiratory system. Aim for optimum breathing rather than maximum breathing, and gradually increase your breath length with practice.

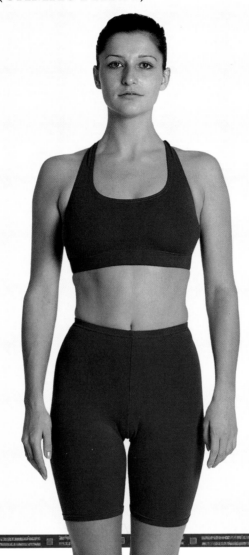

Stand upright, with your feet about 6 inches (15 cm) apart and your hands hanging by your sides. Keep your shoulders back and your chin tucked in. Your pelvis should feel centered and firm, and your weight should be evenly distributed over both feet.

Imagine that you are growing taller— that your neck is growing upward, your chest is getting wider, and your body is opening up. Keep your shoulders, neck, face, and jaw relaxed.

As you inhale, feel as if light is entering you from above and flowing through you to your solar plexus. As you exhale, let the light flood into every cell of your body and nourish it. Breathe in and out five times.

Now feel as you inhale that you are inhaling energy and as you exhale that you are exhaling all toxins and negativity from your system. Spend at least twice as long breathing out as breathing in. If you are breathing in for four seconds breathe out for at least eight seconds.

Because Yoga is a technique of opening up the blockages and balancing the energies in the body, it is essential that a counterpose follows each posture to ensure the flow of energy does not become too strong in the targeted areas of the body. A popular sequence is to start with standing postures, going on to lying on the back, inverted postures and then sitting postures.

After each range of postures there should be a short relaxation session, with a longer period of relaxation to conclude the session. Traditionally, a Yoga session is concluded by readopting Shavasana. Aim to allow at least 10–15 minutes for relaxation after completing an hour's session of Yoga.

Some examples of warming-up exercises are given on pages 48–53, including Salute to the Sun. Some exercises in relation to Yoga and movement are described on pages 68–71 and relaxation techniques on pages 133–5.

VERTICAL STRETCH

Our daily routine, both at home and at work, rarely involves stretching our bodies' muscles in a vertical direction. This often results in poor posture and unbalanced muscle development, and can lead to back pain. The first half of this gentle exercise stretches this much-neglected vertical range of muscles and brings a sense of lightness to the body. The second part is designed to sharpen your awareness of the spine. In returning slowly to the vertical, you are increasing the blood flow to the individual vertebrae. This improves their nourishment and so helps to keep the spine healthy.

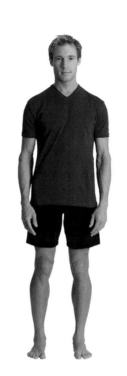

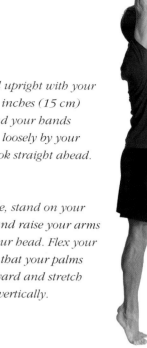

1 *Stand upright with your feet 6 inches (15 cm) apart and your hands hanging loosely by your sides. Look straight ahead.*

2 *Inhale, stand on your toes and raise your arms above your head. Flex your wrists so that your palms face upward and stretch yourself vertically.*

3 *Exhale, and flop down, letting your upper body drop forward from the hips and keeping your knees relaxed or slightly bent. Consciously relax your arms, head, and shoulders.*

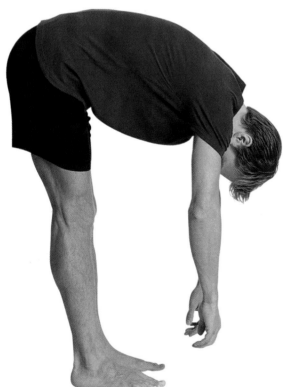

4 *Inhale and come up one vertebra at a time, beginning at the base of the spine, until you have returned to the original standing position. Repeat the complete exercise three times.*

STRETCH WITH FINGER LOCK

This sequence exercises the lungs and so helps to improve your breathing capacity. It also strengthens and tones the muscles of the arms, shoulders, and chest, and helps to alleviate tension in the hands (a part of the body most of us take for granted).

The exercise can be varied by placing the palms together in a prayer position close to the chest and then stretching them upward above the head, keeping the palms together. Reach as high as you can when you inhale, and then bring your hands down to the crown of your head as you exhale. Finally, bring your hands down by your sides.

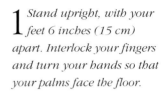

1 Stand upright, with your feet 6 inches (15 cm) apart. Interlock your fingers and turn your hands so that your palms face the floor.

2 Inhale and, locking your elbows, stretch your arms up above your head. Press your palms upward as far as you can, feeling the stretch in your arms and trunk.

3 Exhale, release your fingers, and turn your hands so they are back to back. Slowly lower your arms, keeping them straight at the elbows, until they extend sideways, parallel to the floor.

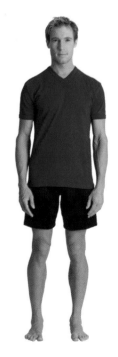

4 Continue to lower your arms in an arc until they are hanging by your sides. Remain standing, relax your body, and breathe naturally, before repeating the sequence three times.

FULL BENDING DOWN (UTTANASANA)

We often bend from the waist, which can strain the lower back. This sequence stretches the leg ligaments (especially the hamstrings) and increases the spine's flexibility, making it natural to bend from the hips. It has the added benefits of trimming the waist, stimulating the nervous system, increasing blood flow to the brain (so soothing the mind), and invigorating the organs.

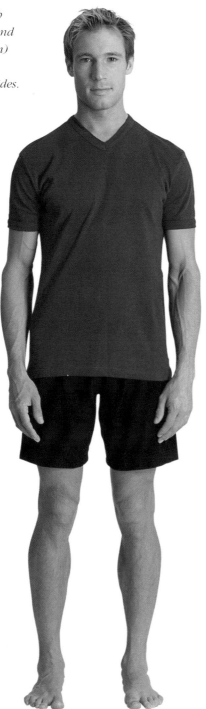

1 *Stand upright, with your feet parallel and about 9 inches (23 cm) apart. Let your hands hang down by your sides. Keep your shoulders back and your chin tucked in.*

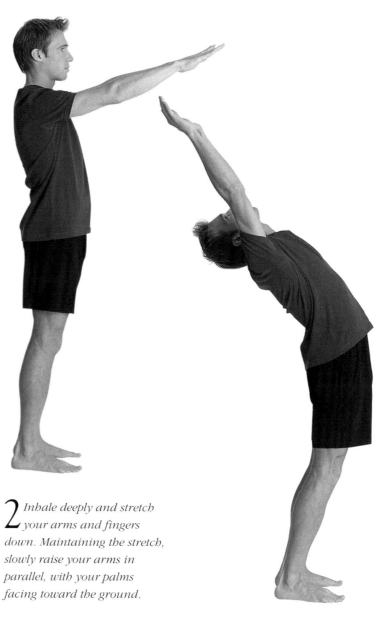

2 *Inhale deeply and stretch your arms and fingers down. Maintaining the stretch, slowly raise your arms in parallel, with your palms facing toward the ground.*

3 *Keep raising your arms until they are stretched high above your head, beside your ears. Arch your body back, with your knees straight, and look up at your hands.*

4 Exhale and, bending from the hips with your arms stretched in front of you, extend your trunk downward. Keeping your knees locked, grasp either your ankles or your shins (depending on how supple you are) with your hands, and press your forehead toward your knees or shins. Try to bring the hips, abdomen, and chest as close to the legs as possible. Relax your head and trunk and breathe normally in this posture for a few moments.

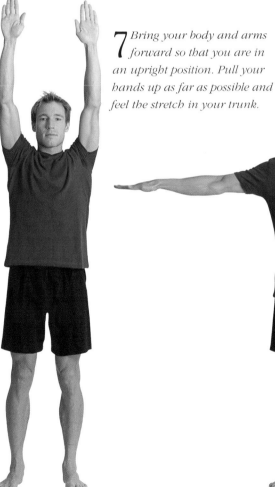

5 Come up slowly, inhaling and raising your arms parallel to your head. Make sure that you keep your arms stretched and your elbows locked.

6 Continue to raise your arms and head together until you are arched back, with your hands above your head. This is the same position as stage 3.

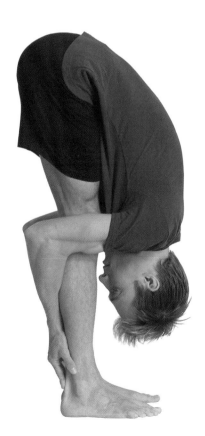

7 Bring your body and arms forward so that you are in an upright position. Pull your hands up as far as possible and feel the stretch in your trunk.

8 Exhale and, elbows locked, gently lower your arms in an arc until they reach your sides.

SALUTE TO THE SUN (SURYA NAMASKAR)

"Salute to the Sun" is traditionally performed at daybreak, facing the Sun, in order to warm up and vitalize the body. If practiced regularly, it increases flexibility, especially of the spine, and helps to improve breathing and blood circulation. (For this reason it should be avoided by those with high blood pressure.) The sequence should be done slowly, using the correct breathing. Repeat it four times, leading on alternate legs, and make sure that you follow each salute with a period of relaxation (see page 133).

1 *Stand upright with your feet together; bring the palms of your hands together in the prayer position. Focus on the breath and the alignment of the body. Think of the rising Sun and its benedictions. Imagine the Sun's rays are penetrating each and every part of your body. Take a few deep breaths in and out, keeping your mind on the Sun.*

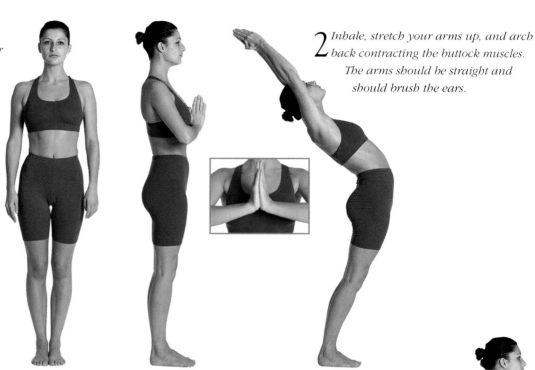

2 *Inhale, stretch your arms up, and arch back contracting the buttock muscles. The arms should be straight and should brush the ears.*

3 *Exhale and bend forward, bringing your head and face close to your knees. Position your hands next to your feet, with your palms facing down and your fingertips in line with your toes. Bend your knees slightly if necessary.*

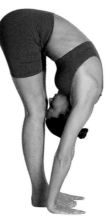

4 *Inhale, draw your right leg backward, and place your right knee on the floor. Your left knee should be bent, and your hands still placed palm down on the floor either side of your left foot. Arch your back and raise your head and chin.*

5 *Hold your breath and take your left leg back so that both feet are together. Keep your arms straight, holding most of your weight on your hands. Your head and body should be held in a straight line.*

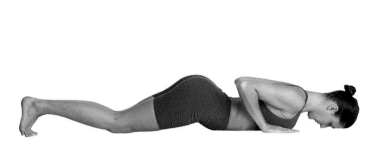

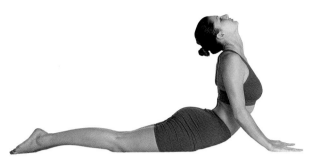

6 *Exhale, bringing your knees and then your chest down to the floor, but keeping your hips raised. Slowly lower your head so that your forehead also touches the floor. The weight of your legs should curl your toes under.*

7 *Inhale, lowering your hips to the floor and point your toes. Without moving the position of your hands, raise your chest and head and arch your neck back. Keep your elbows slightly bent and your shoulders relaxed.*

8 *Exhale, putting pressure on your hands and raising your hips as high as possible. Lower your heels so that your feet are flat on the floor.*

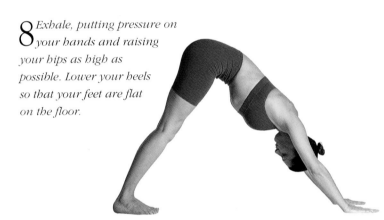

9 *Inhale, putting your right foot forward between your hands. Make sure that the top of your left foot and your left knee are touching the ground. Raise your head and chin so that your body is forming a mirror image of stage 4.*

10 *Exhale, bringing your left leg forward. Keeping your knees straight if possible, bring your head down to the knees as in stage 3. Keep your palms in line with your feet.*

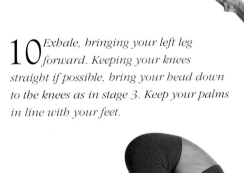

11 *Inhale, stretching your arms forward and up over your head. Arch back as in stage 2.*

12 *Exhale, come up straight, bringing your hands forward into the prayer position. Relax, returning your hands to your sides, and then repeat the whole sequence leading with alternate legs in stages 4 and 9.*

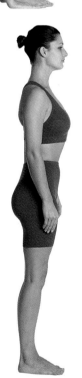

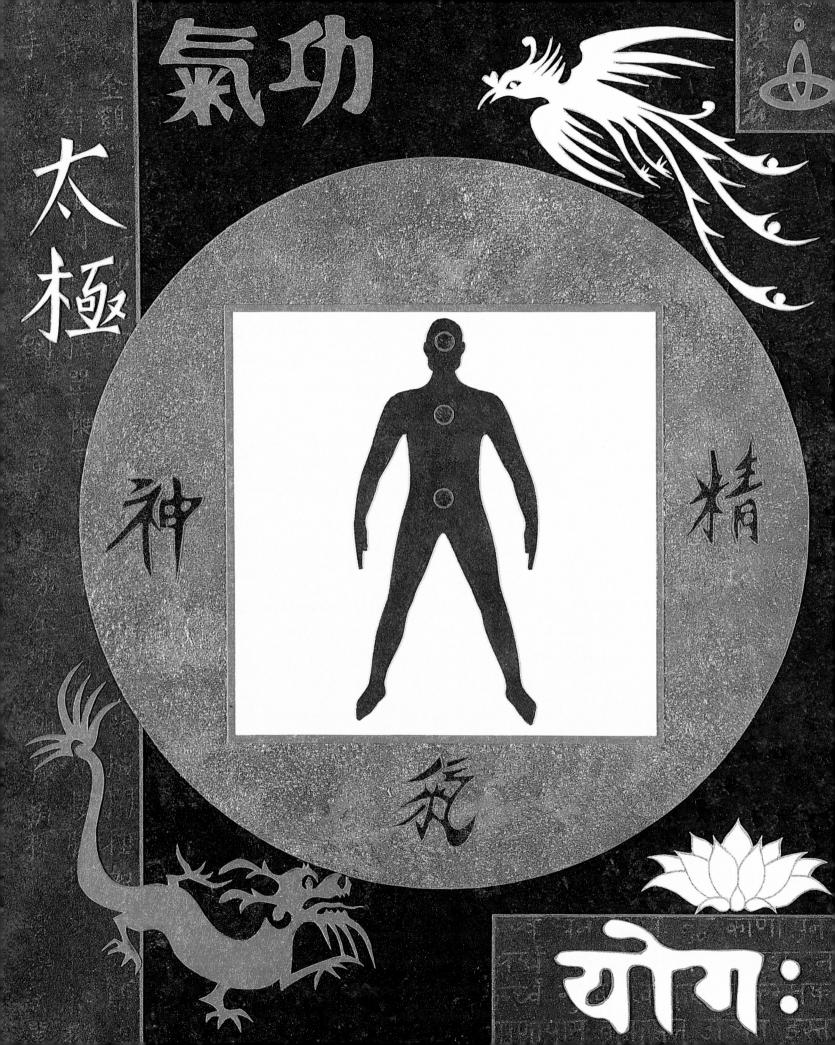

ENERGY, POSTURE, AND MOVEMENT

The human body is designed for movement —something discouraged by many aspects of Western life. Exercise benefits not only the body, but also the mind and emotions. People who exercise regularly recognize its value in enhancing mood, releasing stress, and clearing the mind. Exercising with consciousness of the energies involved can be doubly rewarding— using energy to create more energy.

Cultivating energy need not imply constant effort. We have only to observe an animal such as a cat, which can move from total relaxation to speedy action in an instant. The static postures of Yoga and Qigong are another way of improving the flow of energy. This chapter includes exercises from these disciplines, as well as T'ai Chi, Kinesiology, and dance, to improve your posture, flexibility, and balance.

THE IMPORTANCE OF POSTURE

How people stand, sit, and move can have a profound effect on both their physical well-being and their energy levels. In fact, being self-aware during everyday activities can prove as valuable as following a stringent exercise program. By maintaining poor posture and moving awkwardly we are putting strain on our muscles and bones, and causing energy blockages in our bodies. Conversely, by working in harmony with the energy system we can make any activity easier and more enjoyable, whether it's a walk in the country or a repetitious task such as housework or do-it-yourself jobs.

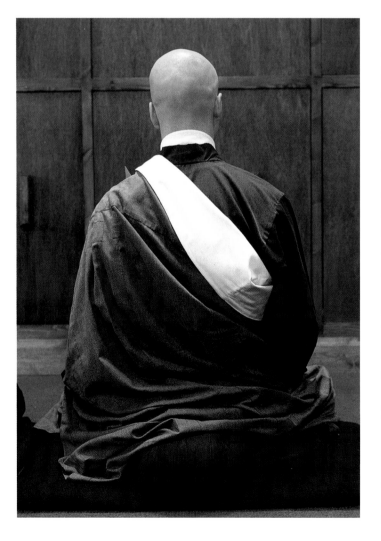

Good posture depends on the spine, which should be lengthened and centered without rigidity or force. It is useful to observe oneself during ordinary, everyday activities, such as waiting for a bus or washing dishes. Many people habitually let their shoulders rise in tension or stand with all their weight resting on one hip and leg, unconsciously throwing their spine out of balance. It is interesting to note that small children hold themselves beautifully, with no conscious effort, but most people lose this natural spontaneity as they grow up, through emotional stresses including anxiety and physical ones such as poor seating at school and work.

Postures often regarded as "relaxed" can actually deplete energy and cause fatigue—slumping on an over-low chair or sofa, for instance, may weaken the lower back muscles and cause stagnation in the lower chakras. At work, crossing the legs or winding them around each other pulls bones and muscles out of alignment. This disrupts both the physical circulation of blood and the flow of energy up the legs and spine and through the two lower chakras. This in turn depletes the energy supply to the higher centers. Holding the telephone receiver between the chin and shoulder twists the neck and jaw. This may block the flow of energy to the throat chakra (which governs communication and listening). It can also lead to quite severe problems in the neck joints.

Maintaining good posture increases your energy levels and helps prevent your muscles and skeleton from being strained. It can also transform your body's silhouette, as standing and sitting correctly tone the abdominal muscles making the stomach look flatter.

To change one's habits requires conscious effort, but has its rewards in lessened tension and greater energy.

When meditating, Buddhists sit in a quiet room, in the lotus posture (see pages 136–7), with open eyes, loose clothing, an upright back, and their breath regulated quietly. This monk is photographed in the temple of Fayuan Si in Beijing.

THE BASICS OF GOOD POSTURE

Good posture can significantly reduce the risk of backache and improve the energy flow in your body. Make sure that you follow the recommended sitting and standing positions, and when getting up use your leg muscles rather than your arms.

Walking enhances the energy flow through all the chakras, and swinging your arms in opposition to your legs (cross-patterning) harmonizes the central nervous system. Try to keep your knees and feet pointing forward, and put your heel down first, exercising your whole foot as the weight shifts to your toes. Thinking of a pole of light up the center of your body lengthens the spine.

If you have to carry heavy objects while walking, holding them close to your body will put the least strain on your spine.

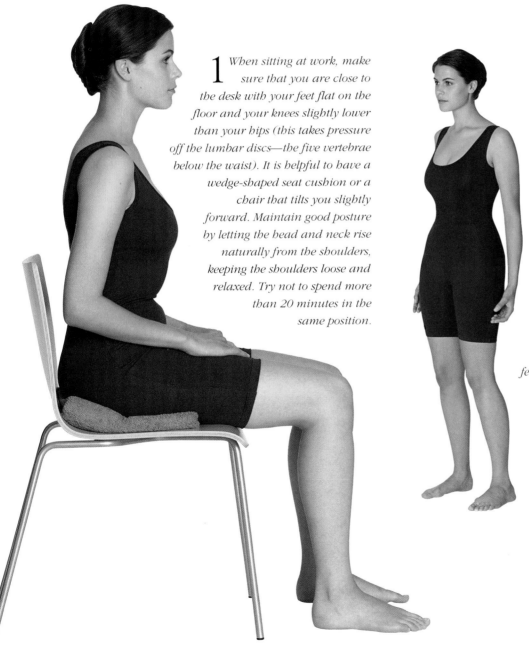

1 *When sitting at work, make sure that you are close to the desk with your feet flat on the floor and your knees slightly lower than your hips (this takes pressure off the lumbar discs—the five vertebrae below the waist). It is helpful to have a wedge-shaped seat cushion or a chair that tilts you slightly forward. Maintain good posture by letting the head and neck rise naturally from the shoulders, keeping the shoulders loose and relaxed. Try not to spend more than 20 minutes in the same position.*

2 *To improve your posture when standing, face a full-length mirror, with your feet pointing forward in line beneath the hip joints. Relax the backs of your knees. Your weight should be in the center of your feet so that your body is tilting neither forward nor backward. Gently draw up your abdominal muscles and feel your tailbone sinking toward the floor. Relax your chest, letting your arms hang loosely and your shoulders drop. If one shoulder is higher than the other (a common fault), gently lower it. Let the head float up on top of the spine. From the side, a straight line should run from the top of your head through your ears, arms, hip joints, and knees to your feet. Your chin should neither be tucked in nor poking forward. There should be a gentle curve in your lower back.*

PHYSICAL THERAPIES

Few adults today are physically perfectly balanced and tension-free. Backache and other muscular and joint problems are rife and are frequently the result of bad posture, repetitive actions (such as prolonged typing) or emotional stress.

Sufferers from chronic pain, tension, or stiffness can benefit from the help of an expert therapist. Massage is good for general tension, while Osteopathy and Chiropractic are excellent for spine and joint problems. They can all benefit the circulation and nervous systems.

Pain or stiffness in any part of the body is reflected in its energy field. Whether or not the therapist works consciously with the energy system (and many nowadays do), releasing physical blockages automatically helps to release blockages in the related chakras. Physically adjusting a painful lower back will therefore restore energy to the lower chakras.

Both Osteopathy and Chiropractic originated in the United States in the 19th century. Although the two disciplines are not identical, they have many similarities.

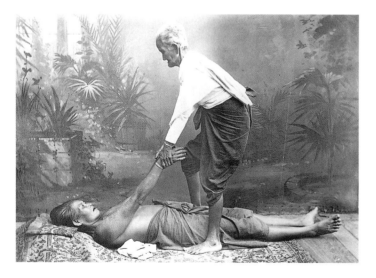

In this photograph, dating between 1900 and 1908, a Thai masseur is manipulating a client. Although Osteopathy and Chiropractic were developed in the West only in the 19th century, massage and manipulation have long been known and practiced in the East.

Both aim to solve mechanical problems in the body through the manipulation of the spine and key joints, together with massage and soft-tissue techniques. The main difference is that Osteopaths consider health largely in terms of the circulatory system, while Chiropractors view it chiefly in terms of the nervous system. Both the circulatory and nervous systems are believed to be impeded by muscle tension or misalignments of bone.

Cranial Osteopathy combines gentle manipulation and simple holding techniques, applied mainly to the skull and sacrum (the five fused vertebrae in the lower part of the back). It is based on the work in the 1930s of an American Osteopath, William Garner Sutherland, who found that the eight bones of the human cranium (skull) are slightly movable, and that disturbance to these bones —during birth or an accident, for example—can affect the functioning of the rest of the body. Sutherland also found that the cerebrospinal fluid that nourishes the brain and spinal cord has rhythms, which relate to the depth and rate of breathing and can be altered through gentle manipulation of the skull. Craniosacral Therapy, recently developed from Cranial Osteopathy, uses similarly gentle techniques to optimize the flow of cerebrospinal fluid and to release traumas to the body/mind system. Practitioners also work in the energy field outside the body. Both techniques are gentle, painless, and relaxing. As well as affording other physical benefits, they improve the flow of energy in the spinal cord.

Because many imbalances become habitual, therapists often recommend clients to maintain improvements by attending movement classes focusing on good posture and balanced movement. In this way, the client will learn to be constantly aware of how his or her body is aligned and will discard bad habits. These classes include Pilates, Body Conditioning, Medau movement, and Feldenkrais. They are all directed at conscious control of postural habits, as is the Alexander Technique, which is not a form of exercise but a re-education in body use.

THE ALEXANDER TECHNIQUE

In the 1920s a Tasmanian actor, F. M. Alexander, regularly lost his voice when performing. By studying himself in mirrors he realized that he was unconsciously contracting his neck and head muscles and needed to relearn their use. Through experimenting on himself, he devised the Alexander Technique, a method of instructing others in the use of their bodies, with particular emphasis on the relationship between the head, neck, and spine.

The technique is usually taught individually. The teacher uses his or her hands to communicate with the client's body, teaching the client to stop bad habits and directing his or her body to stand, sit, lie, and walk correctly. When the head, neck, and spine are in balance, the body feels lighter and energy flows naturally. Stress and tension decrease, and general health improves.

The Alexander Technique does not include specific exercises, but clients are encouraged to spend 15–20 minutes daily lying on the floor, as described below. This is especially useful for postural problems, such as round shoulders or an over-arched lower back, and can help anyone to relax and realign the spine.

1 *Place a book under your head so that it lies at a natural angle. Draw your knees up, with your feet flat on the floor and a hips' width apart. Concentrate on your back relaxing against the floor, the tightness in your neck being released, your chest and shoulders opening out, and your knees floating up toward the ceiling.*

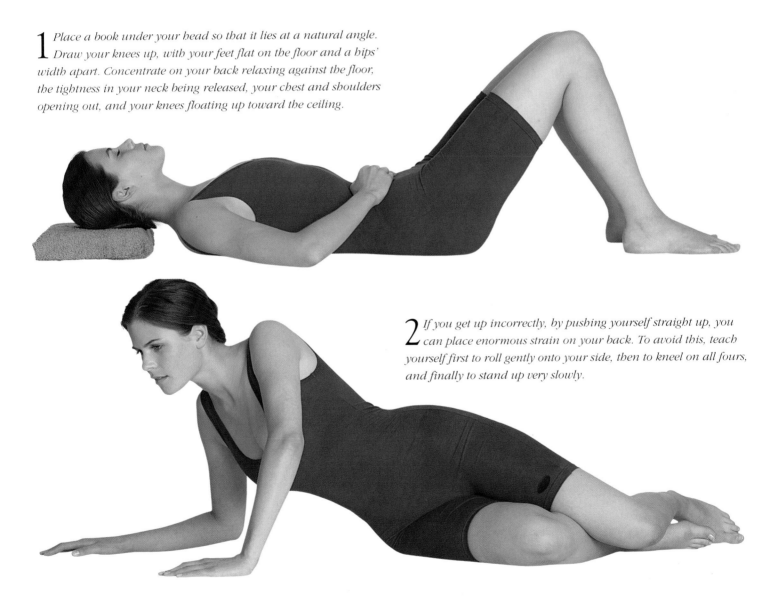

2 *If you get up incorrectly, by pushing yourself straight up, you can place enormous strain on your back. To avoid this, teach yourself first to roll gently onto your side, then to kneel on all fours, and finally to stand up very slowly.*

QIGONG BODY POSITIONING

In Qigong it is vital to hold yourself in a good position in order to maximize the flow of energy or Qi. When you first start Qigong, before your body is used to the practice, it is best to exercise and meditate in a standing position. This enables the Qi to flow more easily. Later, more complicated positions can be taken that concentrate the Qi.

STANDING POSTURE

When meditating in a standing position, you should let the tension go from your shoulders, bend your knees slightly, and keep your feet firmly on the ground, parallel, and about a shoulders' width apart. Relax your behind so that the lower part of your back is smooth, and keep your head erect. One of the most comfortable positions in

One of the major objectives of Qigong is to pacify the mind and spirit. The following positions and movements are intended both to strengthen the flow of Qi through the body and, simultaneously, to allow the mind to rest. Different hand positions are also suggested for meditation, which will benefit various internal organs.

which to meditate is the Qigong basic posture (see page 24), or you can choose one of the three alternatives below. As you meditate, feel as if your whole body is free from restrictions, and let your mind become still and peaceful. All of these standing positions will help you to connect with the energy of the wider universe.

1 *Stand in the basic posture. Raise your hands above your head, with your palms facing forward and your fingers pointing toward the heavens. Relax into the position and feel the energy traveling down your arms and through your body. If the Qi is flowing, you should be able to remain in this posture for a surprisingly long time.*

2 *Stand in the basic posture. Raise your hands above your head, with your palms facing upward. Meditate in this position, feeling as if you are supporting the heavens with your hands.*

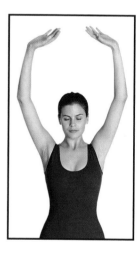

3 *Stand in the basic posture. Slowly raise your arms and extend them outward. Your arms and hands should remain slightly curved as if you are holding an immense ball of energy in front of you. Meditate in this position for as long as is comfortable, feeling as if you are being supported by the energy.*

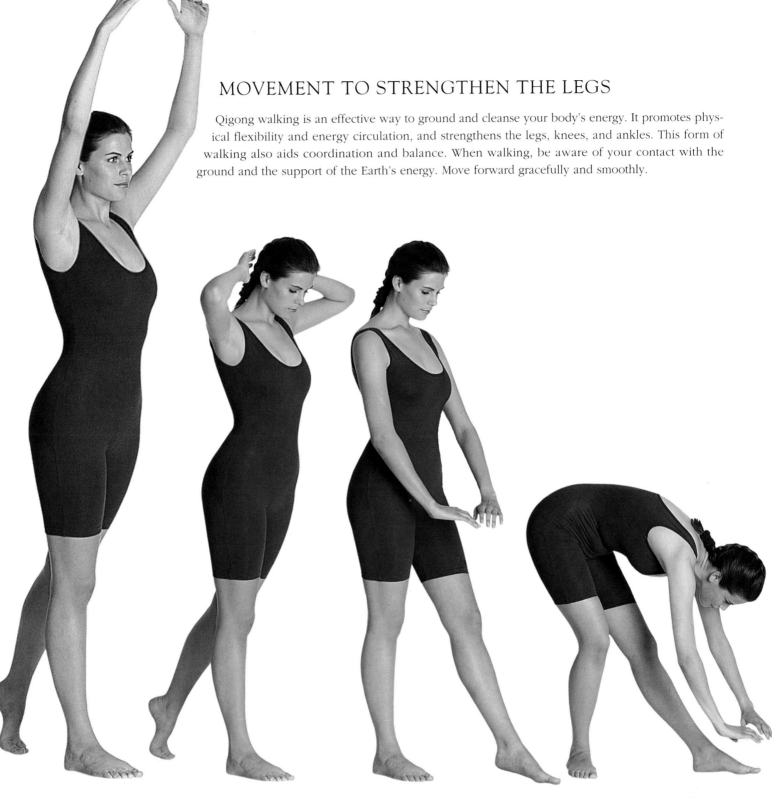

MOVEMENT TO STRENGTHEN THE LEGS

Qigong walking is an effective way to ground and cleanse your body's energy. It promotes physical flexibility and energy circulation, and strengthens the legs, knees, and ankles. This form of walking also aids coordination and balance. When walking, be aware of your contact with the ground and the support of the Earth's energy. Move forward gracefully and smoothly.

1 *Stand with your right foot forward. Raise your hands above your head, curving your arms slightly and keeping your shoulders relaxed.*

2 *Bring your hands down behind your head. Maintaining your weight on your right foot, begin to bring your left foot forward.*

3 *Take your left foot forward and start to transfer your weight to it. At the same time, bring your hands over your shoulders and down your front.*

4 *Push your hands as far as you can down your left leg. Raise your arms, transferring your weight to your back foot. Step forward another ten times.*

SITTING POSTURES

Once the energy is flowing adequately in a standing posture, then a sitting posture can be taken. There are various sitting positions used in Qigong. The key is to take an open gesture and to settle the body down physically. When taking up a position, first slightly stretch and open your body, and then soften and ease off any tension. You should feel supported by the Qi in order to hold the position. Your back should be relatively straight, to encourage the energy to flow through your body, but you should allow the natural curve to remain in your lower back. Your chin should be neither tucked under nor sticking out.

The hand positions suggested can be used in various sitting positions. By placing the hands facing downward, as in position 4,

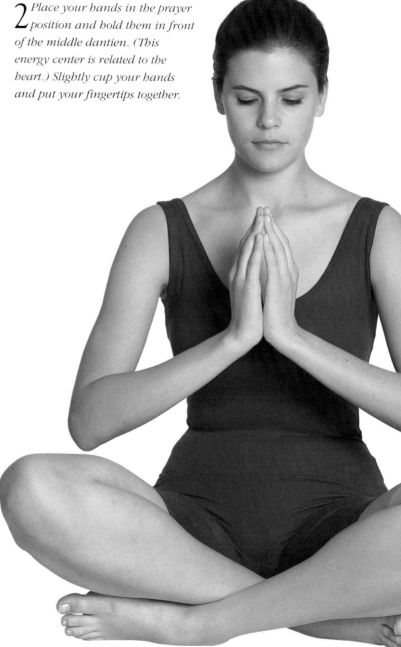

1 Sit on a cushion on the floor, with your legs crossed (men should cross their right leg over their left, and women their left leg over their right). Rest your hands on your knees with the palms facing upward.

2 Place your hands in the prayer position and hold them in front of the middle dantien. (This energy center is related to the heart.) Slightly cup your hands and put your fingertips together.

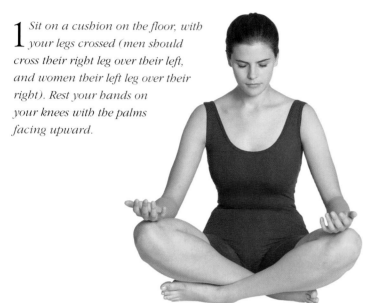

3 Place one hand in front of your upper abdomen with your palm relaxed and facing upward. Bend your other arm at the elbow so that your forearm is vertical. Point your thumb and index finger upward and slightly curl your remaining fingers. This posture represents a drawing of external Qi down from the heavens and a gathering of internal energy around the lower dantien (see page 25).

you are helping to ground the energy. With your hands facing upward you are in a more receptive position. By holding the prayer position you are concentrating Qi in the middle dantien— an energy center in the area of the heart—and by positioning one hand facing forward and the other in front of the upper abdomen, you will sense your chest area opening up.

5 *Sit on one foot with the heel under your perineum. Take the other foot and cross it over the bottom leg, placing the foot as far back as you can. To keep your body in harmony, put one hand on top of the other, in the same order as your legs, and rest them on your knee.*

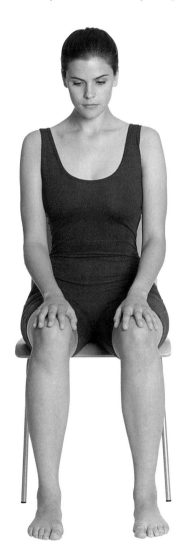

4 *Sit on the edge of a chair, with your head and spine erect, placing your feet parallel and a shoulders' width apart. Place your hands on your knees, with your palms facing down toward the Earth. Feel the opening of your spine.*

T'AI CHI

T'ai Chi translates as the "supreme ultimate." It refers to a system of integrated exercise that employs relaxed breathing, graceful and rhythmical movement, balance, and physical control to improve the circulation of vital energy, or Chi (Qi), in the body, concentrate the mind, and strengthen the spirit. T'ai Chi can really be considered as a form of "moving meditation."

In China there are said to be five "excellences," namely calligraphy, poetry, painting, medicine, and T'ai Chi. A true Master is expected to be accomplished in all five disciplines. Although the movements of T'ai Chi can look slow and even undemanding, adepts show incredible suppleness, agility, relaxation, and mental alertness well into old age.

T'ai Chi exercises are derived from ancient Qigong practice (see page 23), but have been developed extensively in China during the last two centuries. Family groups in different parts of China have created various styles of T'ai Chi, but the general principles of each remain the same.

The key to T'ai Chi is internal, and the focus is placed on the mind and relaxation, rather than on force and strength as in more "external" forms of martial art. As a self-defence system, T'ai Chi training teaches adepts agility, discipline, and flexibility, so that they can repel attackers by reflecting their attack back on themselves.

T'ai Chi consists of solo exercises, paired work known as "Pushing Hands," and movements with weapons. The solo exercises consist of a series of a set number of movements, often 24, which are performed continuously in a slow and rhythmical fashion. The movements can be seen as steps against imaginary opponents, yet the focus

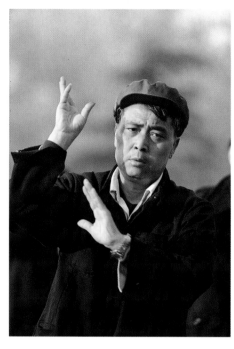

In China, many people practice T'ai Chi outside in the morning (especially under trees) when the external Qi is thought to be most potent and easily absorbed.

is on the internal movement of Qi. The participant should be in a state of relaxation, yet he or she should remain alert.

"Pushing Hands" are exercises of balance and timing, carried out with a partner. These exercises are of great importance in developing skill in T'ai Chi, for they embody the key principles of using softness against hardness, yielding against force, and emptiness against fullness. These principles are summarized in the Yin-Yang symbol, also known as the Great Polarity or T'ai Chi (see page 20). It is said that it is easier to perform these exercises with a child than with a strong opponent because children employ these principles naturally in their movements.

There are three weapons used in T'ai Chi: the sword (*jien*), the one-edged knife or cutlass (*dao*), and the rod or staff (*gan*). The weapons should become an extension of the person's Qi, so that they form an integrated part of the smooth, sequenced movements.

Although it originated in China, T'ai Chi is now taught and practiced throughout the Western world. It is recognized not only as a form of self-defence and a sport, but also as an essential form of exercise for health and healing. Practice is simple as no special equipment is required: only limited time and space are needed, and the movements are accessible to all, regardless of age, sex, or physical ability. It is also a very complete form of exercise, as it not only exercises the limbs and muscles but also improves respiration and cardiovascular function, balances the nervous system, and calms the mind. It has long been recognized that T'ai Chi practitioners often enjoy good health and flexibility well into old age.

WAIST SWINGS

Most T'ai Chi classes nowadays begin with a warm up to loosen the waist and hips. This not only makes it easier to create a rhythmical flow in the body when performing the set series of movements, but also helps to stretch and tone the abdominal muscles and to massage the internal organs.

1 *Stand with your feet a shoulders' width apart, toes forward, knees slightly bent, and arms loosely by your sides. Turn to one side by moving your hips and waist and swinging the hip bone forward. With the momentum from the waist, the arms will swing around.*

2 *Repeat the swing on the opposite side of the body. Keep turning from side to side, making sure that you move from the waist and hips only. The arm swing should arise naturally from the momentum of the movement. Do not try to swing your arms because this breaks the flow. Continue swinging for several minutes until the whole body feels loose and warm.*

STANDING POSE

All T'ai Chi begins with a period of silent standing to calm the mind and unlock energy. This pose can be practiced on its own, building up from a few minutes to longer intervals daily. Although it seems simple, the pose has a powerful effect on the body's energy, increasing stamina and resilience.

Stand with your feet a shoulders' width apart. Your toes should point forward, with your arms and fingers hanging loosely by your sides. Keep your neck and shoulders relaxed.

Check that your spine is straight and imagine that you are being pulled up by a string from the top of the head. The knees should be very slightly bent and not locked.

Draw your chin in a little and look forward and slightly downward with your eyes.

Inhale and exhale gently, allowing the mind to become relaxed, but remaining alert.

Regular practice will build up body stamina and increase mental alertness.

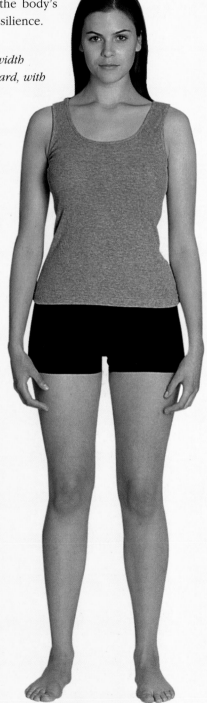

BASIC POSTURES

In T'ai Chi there are eight basic postures. The first four relate to the points of the compass—south, north, east, and west—and the movements of warding off, rolling back, pressing and pushing. The next four relate to the corners of the compass—southeast, northwest, southwest, and northeast—and the movements of pulling, splitting, elbowing, and shouldering.

There are also five "attitudes" that relate to moving forward or backward, left or right, or concentrating on the middle. These correspond to the five elements in Chinese medicine (see page 20). Two of the first four poses can be practiced in sequence to get the feeling of the lightness and flow of T'ai Chi; these are the poses for pressing and pushing.

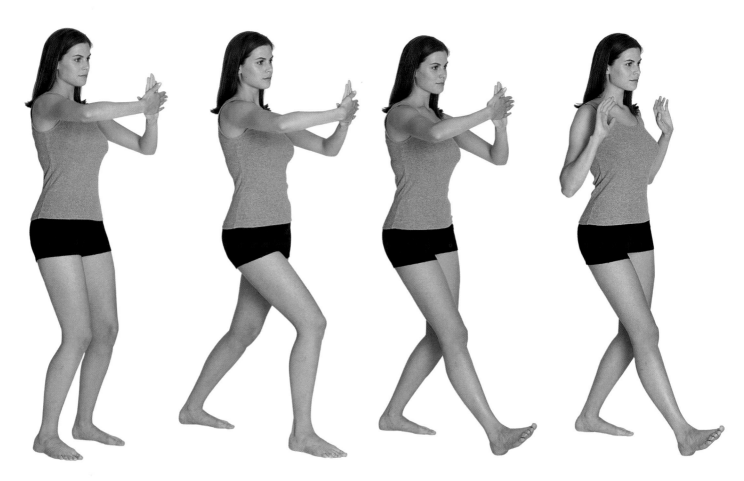

1 Start in the basic standing pose. Inhaling, raise your palms slowly till they are in front of your chest. Hold your right hand parallel to the ground, with the palm facing inward. Place your left hand vertical to the ground, with the palm facing outward. Your two palms should be just touching one another.

2 As you exhale, step forward with your right leg, bending it as you transfer your weight onto it. Your back leg should be stretched, but slightly bent. At the same time, push gently with your left palm. The right palm "resists," but also "yields" and flows forward until the hands are at a shoulders' width distance from the body.

3 Next transfer your weight back onto your rear leg, bending it. Stretch out your front leg (but keep it slightly bent) and rock back on your heel. At the same time gently inhale and pull your right palm toward you. Now it is the left palm that "resists," but also "yields" as it is gently propelled back toward your chest.

4 As the hands reach the chest draw them a shoulders' width apart, with the palms raised in front of you, and slowly complete your inhalation.

Repeat the exercise several times, moving smoothly from one pose to the next. Breathe rhythmically and focus on the flow of energy in the body.

PUSHING HANDS (T'UI SHOU)

Through Pushing Hands all the principles of T'ai Chi can be experienced. After a while you become very sensitive to the movement of energy in both your own and your partner's body and can almost anticipate their movements. This becomes very useful when T'ai Chi is used in self-defence, as it teaches you to anticipate the moves of your opponent and then to dissipate them.

When practicing Pushing Hands, try to sense your partner's state of balance, and even his or her mental state. If you want to, you can close your eyes, but make sure that you remain alert at all times. With experience you will find it easier to detect the moment when your partner is nearest to overbalancing. You should remain in constant contact with your partner throughout this exercise.

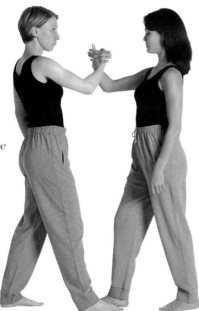

1 *Stand opposite each other with your right legs bent and carrying most of your weight. Your left legs should be extended behind and your right feet level with one another. Touch your right hands lightly together at the wrists, with palms facing your body. Keep your left hands down by your sides for balance.*

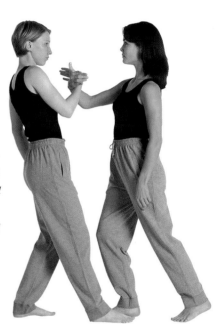

2 *Gently transfer your weight onto your back leg. Bend it a little, and straighten your front leg. At the same time, pull your right hand back and across your torso in a circular movement taking your partner's hand with you. As you "pull," your partner "yields," allowing his or her hand to be drawn to you.*

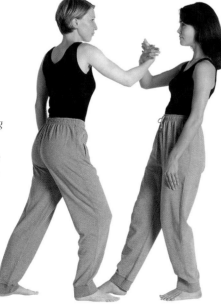

3 *As you finish drawing your partner in, the position begins to reverse itself. Your partner starts to transfer his or her weight onto the back leg and "pulls" inward while you "yield."*

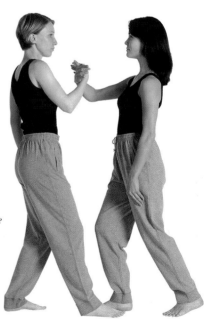

4 *Keep rotating backward and forward for a few minutes, remaining aware of your own and your partner's energy. Repeat the movement, leading with your left legs and with your left wrists now touching.*

YOGA POSTURES

Slouching and generally poor posture can put enormous stress on the lower spine, hips, and pelvis, and can result in backache. Even everyday actions such as carrying a bag on the same shoulder can, over time, cause muscles to become more developed on one side of the body than the other, thereby throwing the whole frame out of alignment. Those who practice Yoga follow a sequence of *asanas* or postures that are designed to work systematically on every part of the body, so that the muscles and skeleton remain healthy and in balance.

TRIANGLE POSE (TRIKONASANA)

The following sequence is a simple version of the Triangle, which is one of the 12 basic Yoga *asanas* (postures) and has a number of variations. This strong lateral stretch has many benefits. It firms the legs and buttock muscles, opens the pelvic region, stretches the inner thighs, and trims the waistline. By toning the abdominal muscles and organs, it can aid digestion and elimination, and by expanding the chest, it helps to increase lung capacity and aids the flow of Prana through the body.

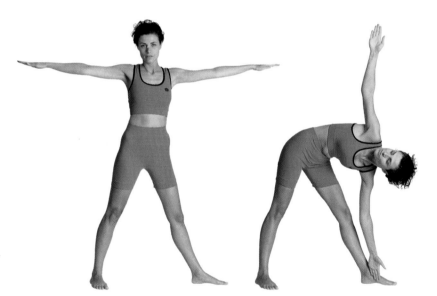
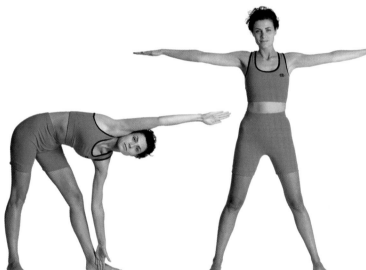

1 *Jump and land with your feet about 3 ft (1 m) apart. Inhale and raise your arms to shoulder level. Stretch them out so they are parallel to the floor, palms facing down. Turn the left foot 90° away from the body, keeping both heels in a straight line. Turn the right foot slightly in toward the left.*

2 *Inhale and, depending on how flexible you are, bring your left hand to your left shin or ankle, or rest it on the floor beside your foot. Lift your right hand straight up so that it is perpendicular to the floor. Turn your neck and look at the palm of your right hand and hold your breath.*

3 *Exhale and, keeping your left hand stationary, pull your right arm down behind your right ear (or touching your ear) so that it is lying parallel to the floor. Look straight ahead. (It is important that your right hand is behind the ear: otherwise there is very little pull on the side muscles.)*

4 *To return to the starting position, inhale and raise your body until you are upright. Make sure that your arms are straight and hold them at shoulder level, parallel to the floor. Exhale, and bring your hands down by your side. Repeat the whole sequence, leading with your right foot.*

SHOULDER STAND (SARVANGASANA)

One of the most popular Yoga *asanas*, the Sanskrit term Sarvangasana means "All Parts Posture." This implies that the Shoulder Stand is good for every part of the body. However, it is particularly good for the thyroid and parathyroid, which are two of the most important glands in the endocrine system.

The Shoulder Stand should not be attempted by people with high blood pressure, chronic back problems, or ailments of the neck, eyes, and ears. Some also advise women to avoid it when pregnant or having a heavy period. Beginners should support their shoulders with a towel.

1 *Lie on your back with your legs straight out, feet together and hands, palms down, by your sides. Inhale and, holding your breath, slowly raise both your legs off the floor pressing down with your hands into the floor. Your knees should be straight, but beginners may find it easier to keep them bent.*

3 *To return to the starting position, tilt your legs over your head at an angle of about 45˚. Stretch your arms out behind your back and place your hands flat on the floor. Slowly, and with control, unroll your body vertebra by vertebra so that your spine and behind are flat on the floor. Then lower your legs to the floor and relax for a short time.*

2 *Raise your legs over your head, supporting your bottom with your hands. Gradually bring your hands down your back so that you are supporting the lower back with the palms of your hands. If comfortable, stretch your legs up so that your whole body is in a vertical position and your chin is pressed into your chest. Pull your elbows in and move your hands closer to your shoulders to further straighten your body.*

If you are not comfortable at first, attempt only the half shoulder stand (as shown). Straighten your legs and keep your hands close to your behind. Relax your feet and legs.

THE FISH (MATSYASANA)

The Fish is the counterpose to the Shoulder Stand and should be practiced after it. It helps release any stiffness in the shoulders and neck caused by doing the Shoulder Stand. Holding the Fish position improves the lungs' breathing capacity, as the rib cage is fully expanded in the posture. It exercises the chest, neck, and back and removes stiffness from the cervical, lumbar, and shoulder muscles. It also strengthens the thyroid and parathyroid glands, which regulate the levels of calcium in the blood.

1 *Lie on your back with your legs straight and your feet together. Place your hands under your thighs with your palms face down and your elbows reasonably close to each other. Your head should be resting gently on the ground.*

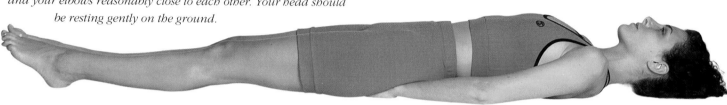

2 *Inhale and, putting pressure on your elbows, raise the upper half of your body so that it is about 45° from the floor. As your elbows bend, keep them tucked under your body. Make sure that your thighs remain flat on your hands and that your legs do not bend, twist outward, or lift from the floor.*

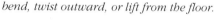
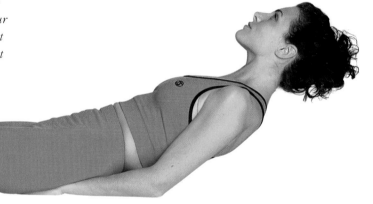

3 *Arch your back, bending your neck as far back as possible. Bring the top of your head back onto the floor, keeping your chest raised above the ground. Take a few deep breaths in and out. To come out of the posture, inhale, put pressure on the elbows and raise your trunk up, release your neck, and bring your back and head gently onto the floor. Release your hands.*

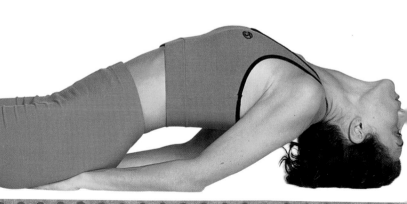

THE COBRA (BHUJANGASANA)

The Cobra is so named because it is said to resemble the snake when its hood is raised. As the spine rolls back, vertebra by vertebra, it helps develop strong back muscles and increase the flexibility of the spine. It also strengthens and tones the abdominal muscles and is said to produce body heat and to help fight infection. In women it tones the ovaries and uterus and can be used to relieve period pain. There are many variations of this posture, which further tone the spine.

1 *Lie face down on the ground with your forehead touching the floor. Bend your arms and place your hands, palms down, directly beneath your shoulders. Put your legs and feet together and point your toes.*

2 *Inhale, and slowly raise your head by first almost touching the ground with your nose, and then with your chin. Now, using your back muscles rather than pushing up with your hands, slowly raise your chest and torso up and back. Make sure that you keep your hips and legs flat on the floor.*

3 *When your arms are almost extended, arch your neck and shoulders back. Hold your breath (or breathe gently) and keep the posture for as long as you comfortably can. Feel the stretch in the whole spine. To come back, exhale and slowly lower your chest and arms, looking straight until your head touches the floor. Lay one hand on the wrist of the other arm and rest your face sideways on your hands. Repeat the sequence three times.*

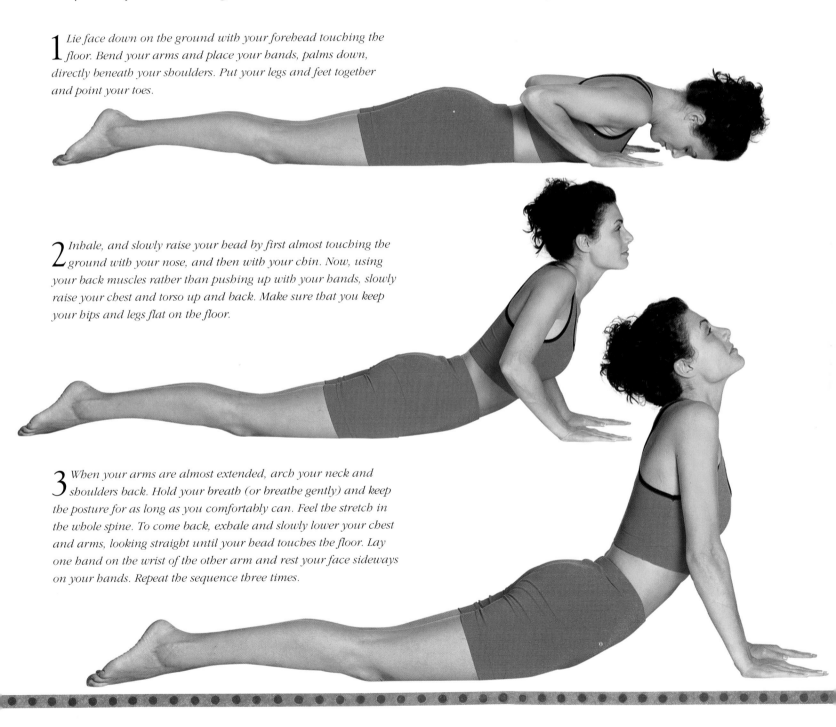

KINESIOLOGY

Good posture is important for a really healthy body. When the spine is straight and has easy movement, the energy, nerve impulses, and blood supply can flow unimpeded to the various organs. Because our skeleton is held in place by muscles, these have to be well balanced if we are to achieve good posture. Kinesiologists test for, and correct, muscle imbalances—by noting which muscles are weak and which are tight—and so are able to restore postural balance.

In order for the body to move effortlessly it needs to be well coordinated. This requires good communication between different parts of the body: the brain and muscles; muscles in relation to each other; the eyes, ears, and speech organs. Through muscle testing, Kinesiologists are able to assess how good or bad a person's co-ordination is, and to recommend exercises that are effective in improving his or her coordination when it is deemed to be necessary.

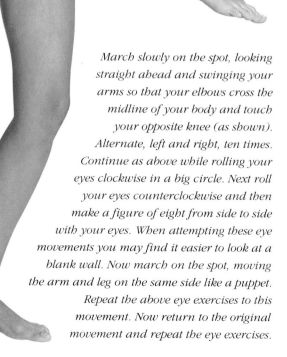

CROSS CRAWL EXERCISE

Cross Crawl, as the name suggests, is an exercise based on a baby's crawling movement. It aims to improve coordination between the right and left sides of the body and the right and left hemispheres of the brain. Although the original research was designed to help brain-damaged children, Kinesiology muscle testing shows that many children and adults who are not brain-damaged can also benefit from exercises to improve their coordination. It has proved to be particularly helpful to those suffering from dyslexia, those who have learning difficulties, or those who are generally clumsy or forgetful.

When we are babies our crawling movements help to develop neurological connections between the right and left hemisphere of our brain and the two sides of our body. These early connections are important for our later development. When both brain hemispheres are activated and working well together as an integrated whole, we function more successfully both in our physical movements and in our thinking.

Many people have found this self-help exercise to be beneficial. If, however, you feel uncomfortable, then stop—it may be that you would find a consultation with a qualified Kinesiologist more rewarding.

March slowly on the spot, looking straight ahead and swinging your arms so that your elbows cross the midline of your body and touch your opposite knee (as shown). Alternate, left and right, ten times. Continue as above while rolling your eyes clockwise in a big circle. Next roll your eyes counterclockwise and then make a figure of eight from side to side with your eyes. When attempting these eye movements you may find it easier to look at a blank wall. Now march on the spot, moving the arm and leg on the same side like a puppet. Repeat the above eye exercises to this movement. Now return to the original movement and repeat the eye exercises.

INTEGRATION EXERCISE

The Integration Exercise involves visualization and movements that simultaneously activate both hemispheres of the brain and both sides of the body. This exercise not only has a centering, balancing effect, but also creates a feeling of deep calm as, on an emotional level, it helps people resolve hidden factors that are causing conflict in their lives. The Integration Exercise may be practiced after the Cross Crawl Exercise to make it more powerful, or it may be done on its own.

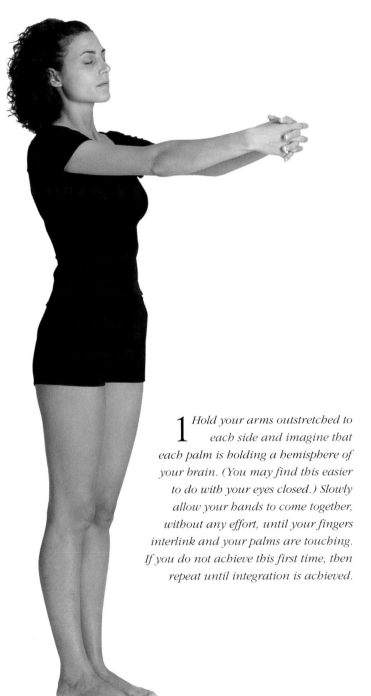

1 *Hold your arms outstretched to each side and imagine that each palm is holding a hemisphere of your brain. (You may find this easier to do with your eyes closed.) Slowly allow your hands to come together, without any effort, until your fingers interlink and your palms are touching. If you do not achieve this first time, then repeat until integration is achieved.*

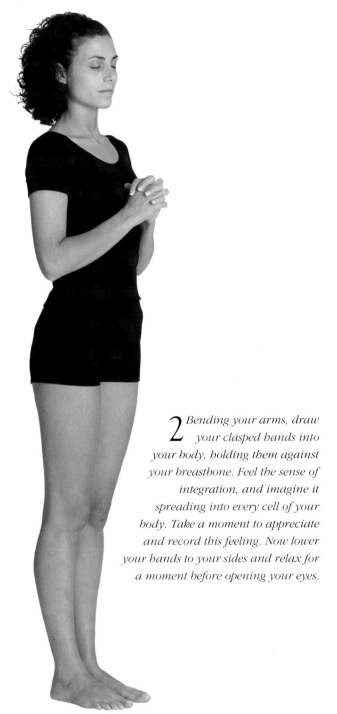

2 *Bending your arms, draw your clasped hands into your body, holding them against your breastbone. Feel the sense of integration, and imagine it spreading into every cell of your body. Take a moment to appreciate and record this feeling. Now lower your hands to your sides and relax for a moment before opening your eyes.*

ENERGY AND EGYPTIAN DANCE

As children we are able to express ourselves through movement without inhibitions long before we are able to talk. It is a method of communication regardless of age or race. However, as adults we sometimes neglect our bodies as vehicles of self-expression.

For years we have looked to the East for methods of healing, spiritual guidance, and ways of relaxation, but dance has rarely been considered in this context. The beauty of dance is that it is an international language that can be used as a means of expressing emotions that move beyond words. Dance is a venting of energy and sometimes may be simply a feeling of pure enjoyment. As Margaret N. H. Doubler observed, "Dance will continue as long as the rhythmic flow of energy operates and until humans cease to respond to the forces of life and the universe. As long as there is life, there will be dance."

Dance is used in many rituals across the world. In the Middle East it occurs at weddings and circumcisions, in South America at baptisms, and in Africa at funerals. Dance in India is perceived as a personal form of prayer. The healing power of dance has long been recognized by tribal communities who have even used it to free the living from possession by evil spirits.

A form of traditional Eastern dance that has recently gained popularity in the West is belly dancing. This is now often known as Egyptian or Middle Eastern dance to avoid the movie-inspired stereotype of a beautiful woman dancing for a fat and aging sultan in a harem! In fact, belly dancing is an ancient art form that originated in the Middle East and Africa. It can be traced down the centuries through art, literature, and mythology. Egyptian tomb paintings dating from the 14th century B.C.E. portray partly-clad dancers whose positions resemble those used

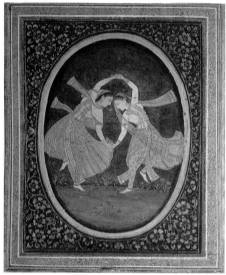

The essential femininity of Middle Eastern dance is evident in this 17th-century Mogul painting of a pair of dancing girls.

in belly dancing. In India, sculptures from the 1st century B.C.E. also have a similarity to belly dance positions.

It seems that belly dance evolved from a combination of rituals and sexual stimulation—the undulating pelvic and abdominal movements were enactments of both conception and birth. During labor and childbirth a woman would squat, bearing down as she rolled her abdomen to assist the birth.

In its new role, belly dancing is a healthy physical art form, which is sensual rather than explicitly sexual in emphasis. Unlike many Western dance forms, in which the energy and center of gravity is placed in the chest area, belly dancing concentrates the energy in the abdominal and pelvic area. This maintains a close connection with the Earth energies through the base chakra, located at the base of the spine, and the sacral chakra at the level of the sacrum. This is the center of sexual and creative energy, a form of which is represented as a coiled serpent, Kundalini (see page 44). Through belly dancing techniques this energy is activated upward through the spine, creating a mental connection with the pineal gland in the head and generating a more spiritual form of energy. The sacral chakra is also connected with watery elements within the body, such as the menstrual flow, seminal fluid, urine, and intestinal fluids, so energizing this chakra can help some physiological problems.

Belly dancing is an enjoyable and healthy way of toning the abdominal muscles, especially after pregnancy. It energizes the internal organs within the pelvic girdle, increases circulation, and balances the hormones. It is an excellent form of therapy for tension and depression, has the effect of enhancing one's sex life in many subtle ways, and is suitable for all ages and sizes.

FIGURES-OF-EIGHT

Figures-of-eight are one of the basic movements in belly dance. They are particularly good for toning the abdominal muscles and keeping the hips and pelvic bones supple.

When practicing a Figure-of-eight, keep your upper body straight and make sure that all the movement comes from the hips. Balance yourself by gracefully extending your arms so that one is above your head and the other is held out to the side.

Stand with your feet directly below your hip joints. Your feet should be kept flat throughout this movement and your knees should be slightly bent. Push your right hip slightly forward and then sweep it to the back. Now, without pausing, do the same movement with your left hip, pushing it forward and then taking it back. Between them, your right and left hips should trace a fluid and continuous horizontal figures-of-eight.

HIP DROPS

Another basic movement, Hip Drops act on one leg at a time. Regular practice will keep the pelvis supple and help tone your hips, thighs, and buttocks. Although at first it may feel easier to put your hands on your hips, when practicing you should hold your arms in a similar way to the previous exercise. Keep your neck and shoulders relaxed.

1 *Stand upright with your feet placed slightly apart. Place your right foot a fraction ahead of the left. Raise your right heel, keeping your toes firmly on the ground. Keep the knee of your left, supporting leg slightly flexed; do not lock it. Using the toes of your right foot as a platform to push from, lift your right hip at the side, bring the hip forward, and drop it.*

2 *Now take your right hip in an arc from the front to the back and drop it in the back position. Lift the hip and reverse the movement, taking the hip to the front again. The complete movement should be rhythmic and bouncy. After several forward and back drops with the right hip, repeat the movement on the left side of the body.*

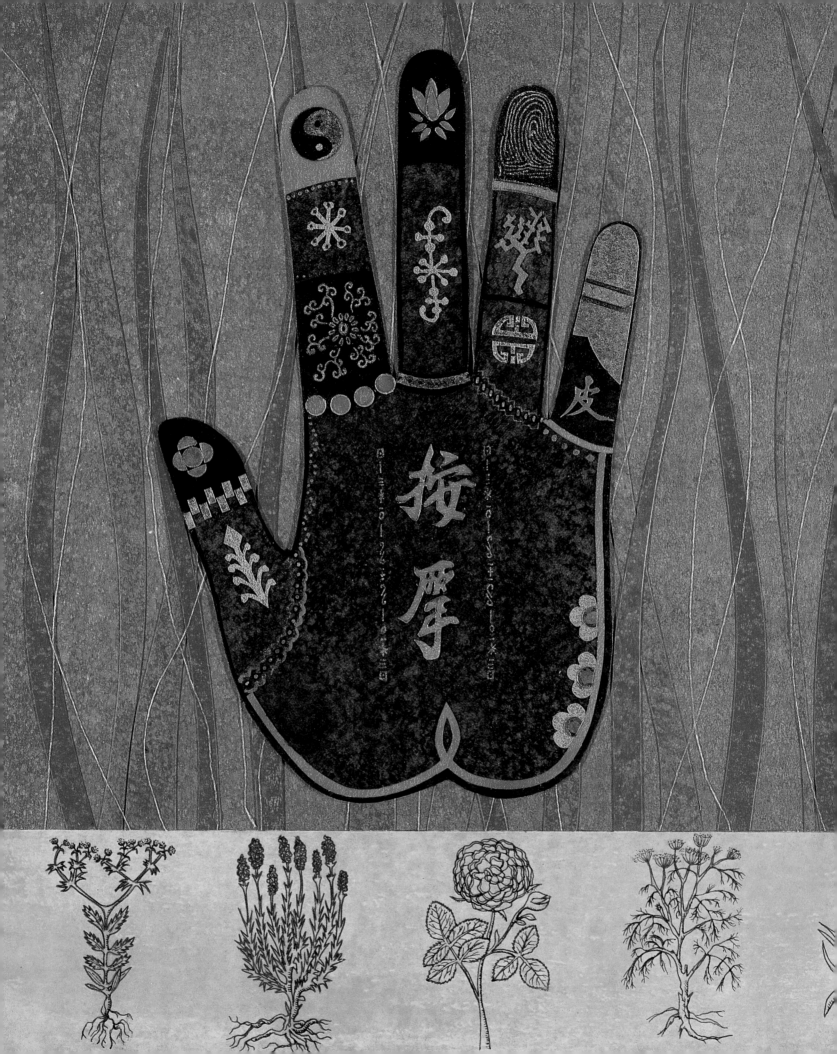

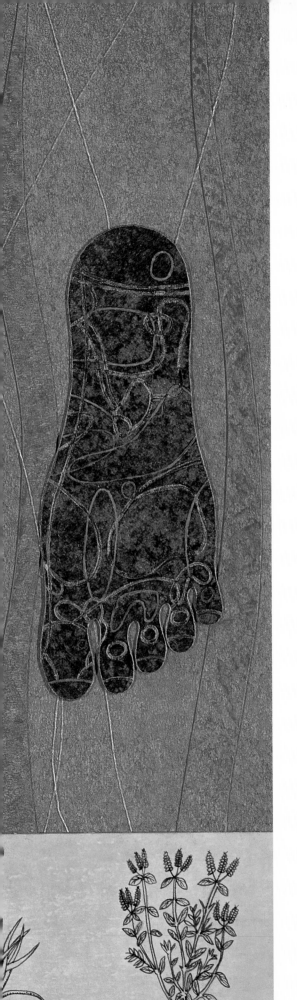

ENERGY, MASSAGE, AND TOUCH

Most theories about energy, whether propounded by the ancient Greeks or modern physicists, make no distinction between the essential energy within humans and that possessed by other life forms. Hippocrates, the father of Western medicine, believed that the same vital force flows through all things. According to Plato's *Phaedrus*, Hippocrates regarded the body as a whole organism, rather than a collection of independent parts, so that a change in one part affects all the other parts. In accepting this concept of an all-embracing nature, we may begin to understand how awareness of our own energy helps us to link with that of other people, plants, and animals. This belief is fundamental to the sensory disciplines of Energy Massage, Aromatherapy, and Reflexology.

PREPARING FOR AN ENERGY MASSAGE

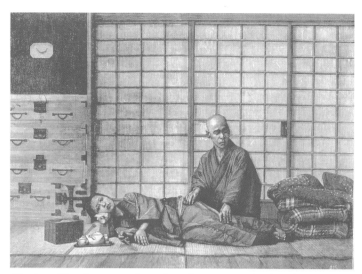

The benefits of massage have long been recognized in the East, where it is part of family life as well as a professional therapy. This Japanese etching shows a masseur working on a woman's leg.

An Energy Massage not only affects the physical body but also changes the levels of energy flowing through the subtle body (see pages 44–5). When giving an Energy Massage, you form a single energy circuit with your partner, merging your fields. The basic aim is to encourage an even flow of energy in your partner, by increasing energy where it is deficient and reducing energy where it is in excess, without imposing your will on the natural energy flow of your partner.

When working with energy make sure that you are properly grounded, in order to feel the supporting power of the Earth. You should be relaxed (so that your own energy is able to flow freely) and aware of the polarity of your hands and of the state of two chakras in particular: the sacrum center for strength and the heart center for compassion.

It is important to know what your own energy is doing when embarking on energy work, so that you do not assume that your partner is the sole source of any impressions you receive from this shared circuit. At first you should focus on yourself more than on the person receiving the massage. This is because, in energy work,

you use your responses and sensations to build up an energy picture of your partner.

To become aware of your own energy field, practice an exercise recommended by Julie Henderson in *The Lover Within*. Stand alone in a room and fill it with your energy, perhaps by moving, dancing, and making sounds. When your energy fills the room, like a balloon squashed into a box, bring it back around your body. Notice how this feels and be aware of where the edges of your energy field are. Is it evenly distributed, or perhaps stronger at the front than at the back, or at the top than at the bottom? Does it reach your feet? Is your field dense or diffuse? Are the edges clear or fuzzy? Does it move or change? Now bounce the edges of your energy field in and out a few times, creating a slight pulsation.

Repeat the whole exercise, noticing any differences the second time. If you wish, extend your energy field out of the room and bounce the edges in and out. Bring it back in, again noticing any differences in feeling. Repeat this exercise daily for a few days.

It is also useful to perform with a friend the T'ai Chi exercise "Pushing Hands," which appears on page 67. This will help you become aware of the positive and negative polarity of your hands, and will encourage an awareness of the energy fields of you and your friend.

You need to work in a warm room, wearing light clothing, and with extra towels or blankets to cover your friend—feeling cold is a serious impediment to the flow of energy. Working on the floor is fine for most people; put your friend on a futon or quilt for comfort. If you have a massage couch it should come up to the level of your groin; if higher, it will be difficult to relax your shoulders, if lower, you may strain your back. Have a couple of extra pillows of different thicknesses handy as many people need extra support under their chest or ankles, lower back or knees. Have your oil handy, ready-blended (see page 89) in a squeezy bottle to avoid spills, and remember that natural oils can smell rancid on the towels unless you wash them in very hot water.

BASIC MASSAGE STROKES

The following basic strokes are described both in terms of their physical purpose and for their particular use when doing energy work. Take care of your posture when giving a massage: keep your back straight and your shoulders relaxed.

EFFLEURAGE OR STROKING

This is normally used in massage to oil the area smoothly, to introduce yourself to the body part you are working on, to learn its contours, to soothe, and to establish a rhythm.

In energy work effleurage is used for sensing a picture of the energy of the body part concerned. Because it is calming for both receiver and giver, effleurage allows the energy fields of both to relax and expand. It is also used for soothing and "closing down" the area after it has been massaged.

Oil your hands and put them on the part you intend to massage at its farthest point from the heart. Your fingers should face in opposite directions, with your hands either side by side or, on a limb, one above the other. Mould your hands to the body surface and stroke, gently but firmly, up the body part as far as you can go. Lightly fan out your hands and draw them back down to the starting point. Repeat several times, re-oiling your hands if necessary, and covering all of the body part you are massaging.

PETRISSAGE OR KNEADING

This stroke is normally used in massage to break up particular areas of muscular tension. In energy work petrissage can be useful for dispersing areas of dense congested energy. This is often linked to muscular tension, but not always, so you can knead deeply or gently, as required.

THUMB GLIDES

These are used normally in massage as alternate thumb strokes, to work deeply into the tissues, always longitudinally along a muscle, and usually on the back. The thumb glide is the main stroke used in energy work for penetrating, connecting up lines of energy (the meridians), and rebalancing.

Face the body part you want to work on, with your hands in the same direction. Pick up the flesh of the body part between fingers and thumb of one hand, squeeze and release it, then repeat with the other hand. Work up and down the body part several times, covering the whole area thoroughly.

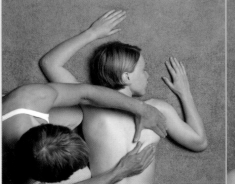

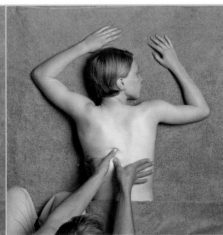

Stand by your partner's back, facing his or her head. Use short strokes up the muscle on the near side of the spine with first one thumb then the other. When you have worked up one side of the back, move to the other side of the body and repeat.

AN ENERGY MASSAGE

This section describes a full body massage, beginning on the back of the legs and working up the back to the neck, then down the arms and abdomen. It finishes on the front of the legs and feet. Vary this routine to suit your partner's requirements or your own preferences: what is important is how you bring awareness into the massage.

When giving a massage, make sure that you remain grounded, relaxed, and in touch with your responses and sensations. Keep your "awareness bubble" wide and be aware of the rhythm of your own breath and that of your partner. This ensures that your massage session is unique, sensitive, and creative.

MAKING CONTACT

Although you can start your massage anywhere on the body, most people feel safer exposing either their backs or the backs of their legs until they relax. As you oil your hands, be aware of your energy field around you. Extend this awareness to your partner's body, from head to toes, and your energy field will naturally move with it to enclose you both in an "awareness bubble."

Make contact by "floating" your hands gently down to the soles of your partner's feet. Hold them for a second, as you become aware of your own feet and their contact with the ground.

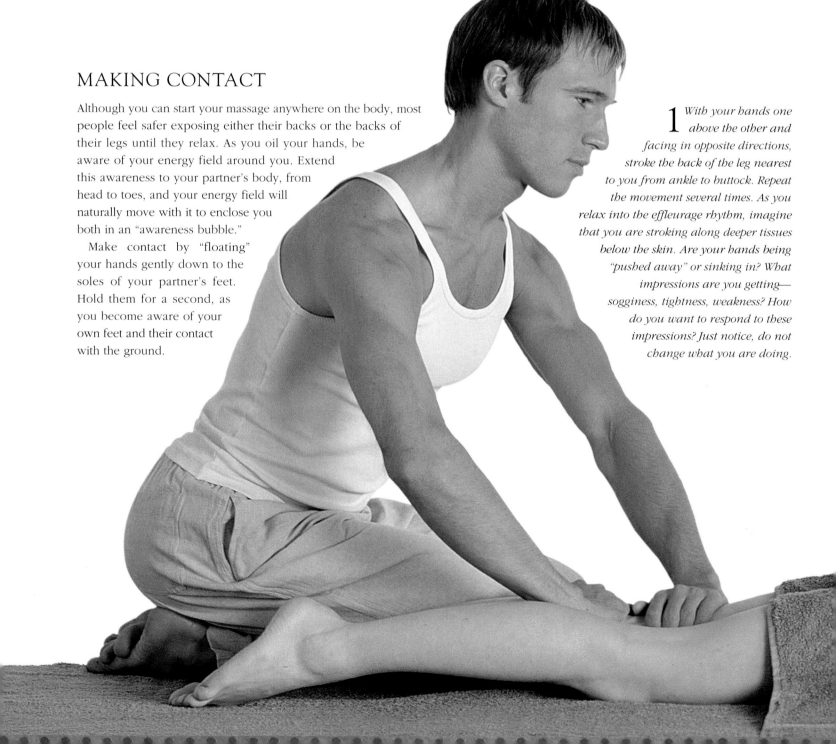

1 *With your hands one above the other and facing in opposite directions, stroke the back of the leg nearest to you from ankle to buttock. Repeat the movement several times. As you relax into the effleurage rhythm, imagine that you are stroking along deeper tissues below the skin. Are your hands being "pushed away" or sinking in? What impressions are you getting— sogginess, tightness, weakness? How do you want to respond to these impressions? Just notice, do not change what you are doing.*

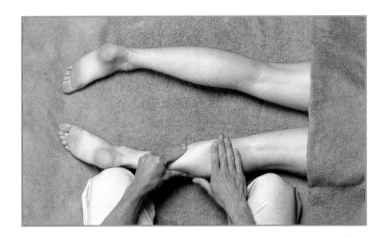
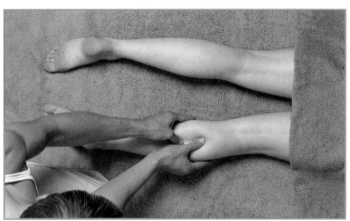

2 *Having thoroughly warmed and relaxed the leg muscles using effleurage, change your stance to face your partner's leg. Knead up the back of the leg from ankle to buttock, rhythmically lifting and squeezing the flesh with alternate hands. Make sure that you maintain close contact with the leg—it is not necessary for you to remove your hands completely from your partner's body between each petrissage stroke.*

Because the surface area varies dramatically as you travel up the leg, you will need to adapt your stroke: make tiny movements with one finger and thumb on the Achilles tendon, and then use the whole of your hands on the calf. The upper leg will need three journeys up and down to cover the inside, middle, and outside of the thigh. Notice the elasticity of the tissues in different areas and how it varies. Knead slowly and deeply on the weak or soft areas of the leg, but work faster and more vigorously on tight areas.

3 *Turn to face your partner's body. Wrap your hands each side of the leg nearest to you. Lean slightly into your thumbs as you glide first one and then the other up the midline of the back of the leg, using short firm strokes and directing your focus down toward the ground.*

Be aware of areas that "let you in," and lean your body weight in to increase your pressure slightly. At the same time, imagine that you have lasers on the ends of your thumbs that are penetrating through to the front of your partner's leg. How deeply can these lasers go in? Do they sink into what seem like troughs or holes? Slow down when they do. Do you encounter slopes or hills? Try and push the hills up the leg with your thumbs to flatten them. We are not talking about the physical contours of the leg here, but rather about the energy contours that you can feel when you imagine penetrating below the surface.

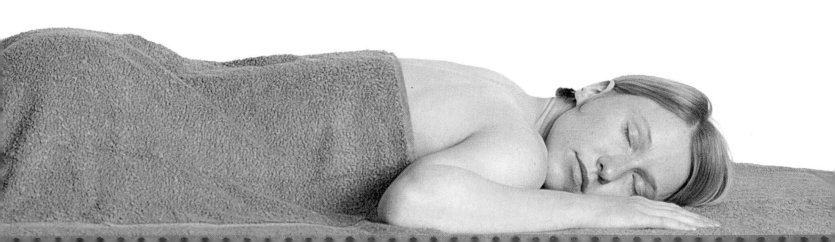

USING POLARITY TO HELP YOU TUNE IN

One of the best ways to encourage your partner's energy to rebalance itself is to create a positive and a negative pole by using your hands in different ways. This is effective anywhere on the body, but the best place to practice it if you are a beginner is on the legs and back.

Using your awareness for both receiving (negative pole) and projecting (positive pole) helps encourage the flow of energy in your partner's body. The increased flow of energy in the legs will ground and refresh him or her. You don't have to "do" very much; just follow the sensations of hills and valleys you feel as you move

up the leg. Observe your own sensations of well-being, too. If it feels good to be in a certain area, linger there. If it feels uncomfortable to be in another, move away from it.

Finish working on this leg with a concluding effleurage in which you relax your focus and simply rhythmically soothe the leg. Move over to your partner's other side and repeat everything on the other leg. Remember that it is likely to feel different on this side, not only because of possible differences in the energy of your partner's legs but also because of your own "polarity preference" in the way that you use your hands.

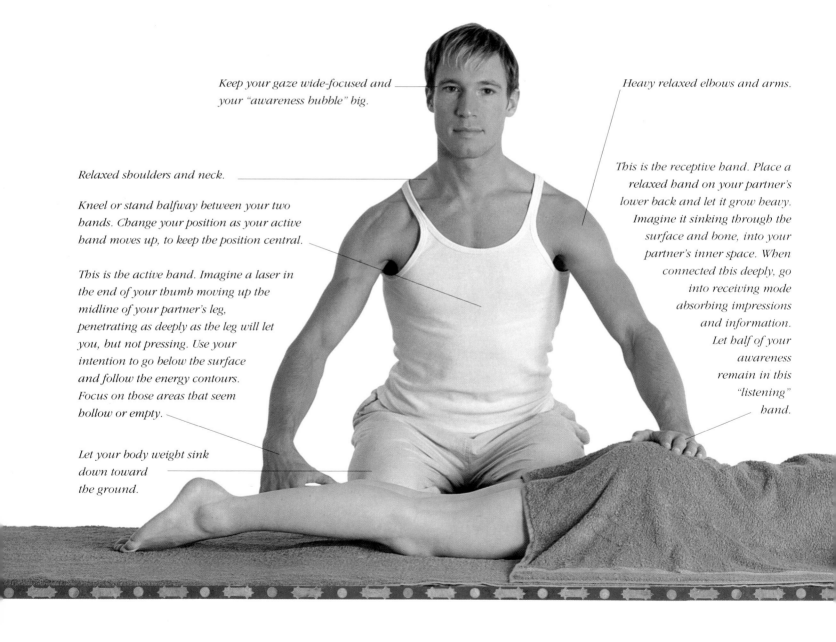

Keep your gaze wide-focused and your "awareness bubble" big.

Heavy relaxed elbows and arms.

Relaxed shoulders and neck.

Kneel or stand halfway between your two hands. Change your position as your active hand moves up, to keep the position central.

This is the active hand. Imagine a laser in the end of your thumb moving up the midline of your partner's leg, penetrating as deeply as the leg will let you, but not pressing. Use your intention to go below the surface and follow the energy contours. Focus on those areas that seem hollow or empty.

Let your body weight sink down toward the ground.

This is the receptive hand. Place a relaxed hand on your partner's lower back and let it grow heavy. Imagine it sinking through the surface and bone, into your partner's inner space. When connected this deeply, go into receiving mode absorbing impressions and information. Let half of your awareness remain in this "listening" hand.

THE POWER OF INTENTION

Once you have been able to tune into the energy flowing through your partner's body, you can learn to uncover the "valleys" (where energy is deficient) and the "hills" (where it is in excess). Then you can use your "intention" to cut through the body like a knife through butter. Work deeply into the valleys. As you penetrate and open up these neglected or deficient areas, excess energy that has been stored in the "hills" will flow automatically into the "valleys," thus restoring the body's natural balance.

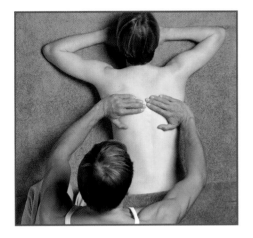

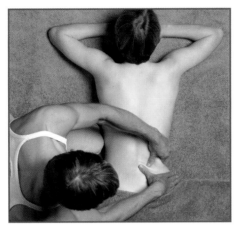

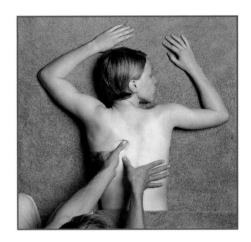

1 *Move up your partner's back. Facing his or her head, stroke gently, but firmly, up the back from the hips. Fan your hands out at shoulder level and draw them lightly down the sides of the back to begin again at the base of the back. Repeat several times, and as you relax into the rhythm of the stroke, notice what impressions and sensations come to you.*

2 *Turn to face your partner's back and knead the whole surface—from the hips up to the shoulders on one side, then back down to the hips on the other. Cover the back two or three times; you will easily notice the congested or "bunchy" areas. By contrast the weak or deficient areas are harder to perceive. However, the latter are much easier to work with in energy terms.*

3 *Glide up one side of the back with alternate thumbs, then switch to the other side. Imagine that you have lasers emitting from the end of your thumbs and penetrating through to the front of your partner's body. Work slowly enough to sense the hills and valleys of his or her energy field, taking note of any impressions or sensations that you receive.*

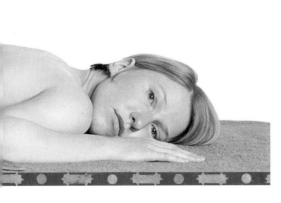

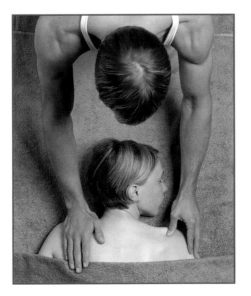

4 *Move behind your partner's head. Place your partner's arms by his or her sides. Lay a receptive hand on one shoulder and place your other thumb on the top of the other shoulder, as close to the neck as you can. Lean into the thumb and slowly glide it along the top of the shoulder. Let the rest of your hand move with the thumb in contact with the shoulder.*

When you reach the joint, repeat the process a little further down the shoulder, angling your pressure slightly more to the front of the body. Repeat again, a little lower still. Then change hands and work on the other shoulder. Conclude with effleurage to soothe the back as before.

MAKING CHANGES

Because energy flows naturally between the neck, chest, and arms, massaging these areas may initially prove difficult but can be deeply rewarding to both you and your partner. You will probably find it easier to connect with your partner's energy through his or her hands. Although many people initially feel vulnerable when exposing their abdomen, it is an area where energy changes can be most easily felt and made. If you work with sensitivity to what you feel, your partner will feel deeply relaxed after the massage.

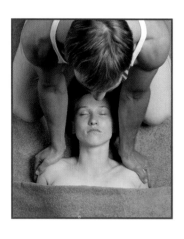

1 *First move any long hair out of the way. Place your hands facing each other on your partner's upper chest. Immediately fan them out over the shoulder joint, then draw them across the back of your partner's shoulders and up the back of his or her neck. Raise your hands and start again. Repeat this modified form of effleurage several times.*

2 *Keep your fingertips at the back of your partner's neck, where it joins the skull, and cup the back of his or her head in your hands. Take care not to lift it too high off the mat or couch. (If you are on the floor, it is easiest to do this kneeling with your thighs on each side of your partner's head.) Curl your fingers and lean slightly back, tuning into the elasticity of your partner's neck as the head moves back a little with you. Repeat the movement rhythmically several times, releasing a little more of your partner's spine each time. With practice, you should be able to see your partner's feet move slightly as you stretch his or her neck. Conclude with more effleurage to the chest and neck.*

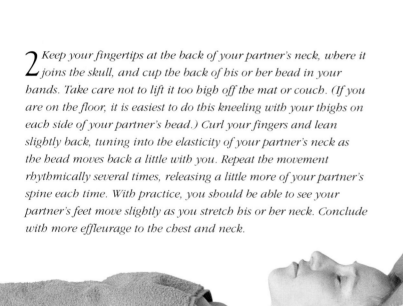

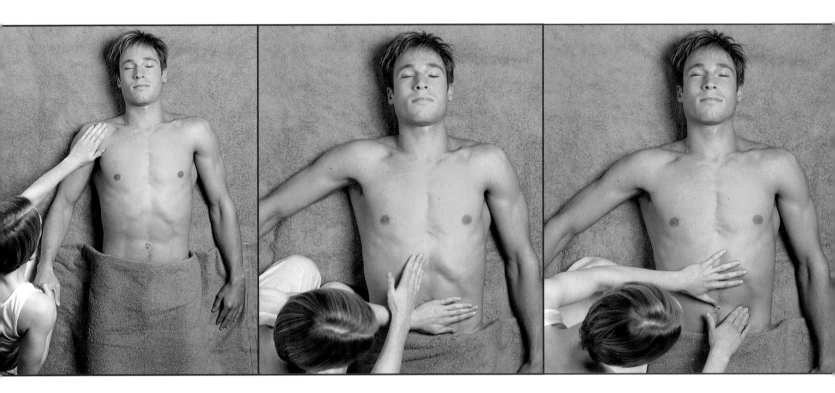

3 Hold your partner's hand as if you were shaking hands. Stroke upward along a part of the arm that you can easily reach with the other hand, and bring the hand down again another way. Now swap hands, changing the position of your partner's arm so that as you stroke up and down you cover a different surface. Keep alternating your supporting and stroking hands in this way until you have covered all the arm.

Stretch your partner's palm open with your thumbs, using your fingers to support the back of his or her hand. Make small circular movements with your thumbs all over the palm. Then, supporting your partner's wrist with one hand, hold the sides of his or her little finger at its base between the thumb and index finger of your other hand. Slide up the finger, leaning your body back to stretch the finger and arm. Repeat on all the other fingers and both thumbs.

4 The abdomen is the area where energy changes can be felt most easily. Start to work on this region by resting both hands on your partner's abdomen. Ground yourself and tune in to your partner's energy again before you start working on this vulnerable area. Oil the abdomen, making circular strokes in a clockwise direction with one relaxed hand around the navel area. Let your other hand join in when you feel ready so that both your hands are stroking rhythmically around the center of the abdomen. Continue for a minute, or longer if your partner likes it. Remember to keep your shoulders down and your arms and hands relaxed.

5 Rest a "listening" hand on your partner's upper abdomen. Place the flattened fingers of the other hand on the side of the lower abdomen, next to your partner's hip bone. Applying slow, gradual pressure and "listening" for any sign of resistance, lean some body weight in and project energy down as deep as you can into your partner's inner space. If you sense feelings of resistance, stop applying the pressure. Only go as deep as your partner will allow, and remove the pressure as slowly and gradually as you applied it.

Moving your "listening" hand around as necessary, continue these pressures in a diminishing spiral on the abdomen until you have almost reached the navel, which should not be pressed. Pay attention to the areas of deepest penetration; stay in each with still and relaxed attentiveness until you feel something change. Never push or force, and make sure that you remain grounded and aware of your breathing.

GROUNDING YOUR PARTNER, CONCLUDING, AND SEPARATING

The lower limbs physically support the rest of the body. Improving the flow of energy through the thighs, knees, calves, ankles, and feet creates a stable foundation for the body. It also increases awareness of the supporting power of the Earth, "grounding" your partner and anchoring him or her in this security. Massaging and holding your partner's lower limbs will bring warmth and relaxation to his or her legs and feet, to create a sense of balance within his or her body.

It is important to complete the Energy Massage carefully and deliberately. Allow both yourself and your partner time to absorb the changes and benefits of the session, before separating from each other emotionally, energetically, and physically.

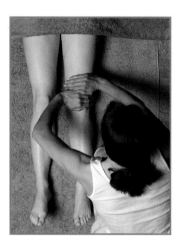 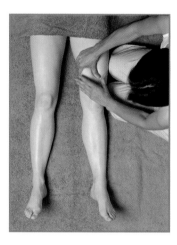

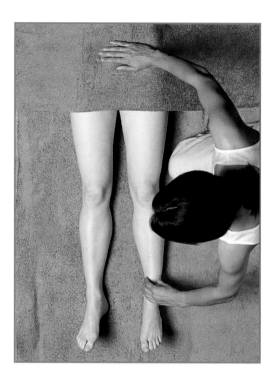

1 *Apply effleurage to the front of the leg in the same way that you did to the back (see page 83). Start at the ankle and work upward, adding a little extra to the stroke on the outside of the thigh—which is higher than the groin—and stopping slightly short of the groin on the inner thigh. Repeat enough times to get a rhythm, remembering to keep your shoulders down during this long stretch.*

2 *Divide the thigh into three sections (front and two sides). Using petrissage (see page 79), cover each section, staying sensitive to possible tender areas. You will find that you can knead the inside of the knee, the kneecap itself and the area just above it. Energy structures are often distorted around the knee, so you may discover troughs and hollows in this area, as well as hills or congested areas.*

3 *With a "listening" hand on the abdomen, glide up the front of your partner's leg from the ankle to the top of the thigh. The thumb of the other hand should go around the kneecap. Keep the rest of your hand in light contact with your partner's leg, and direct your intention downward through to the back of the leg.*

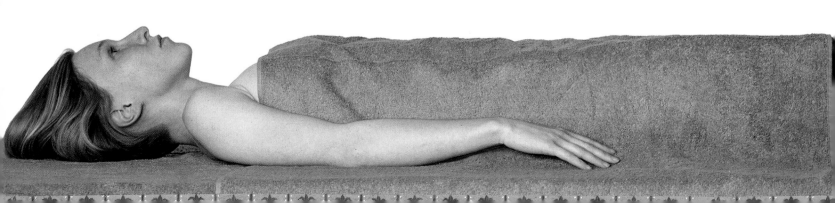

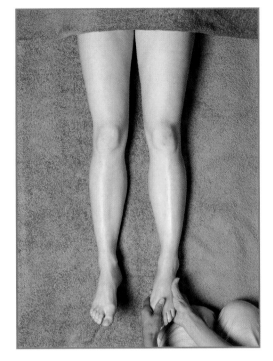

5 *Hold the base of your partner's big toe at the sides between your thumb and index finger. Slide up the toe as you lean backward to stretch it. Repeat on all the toes in turn. Imagine strings going from each toe right up into your partner's body and stretch the strings as you stretch the toes. Now repeat stages 1 to 4 on the other leg.*

4 *With one hand, support the foot of the leg you have been working on under the ankle. Using the thumb of the other hand, glide down the top of the foot between the tendons, from ankle to toes, while your fingers move along the sole. Angle your thumb and fingers toward each other, imagining that the "lasers" on each are meeting in the middle of the foot. Work slowly and deeply, paying attention to hollows.*

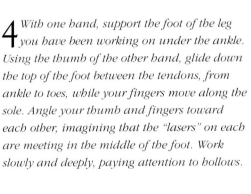

CONCLUSION
Hold both your partner's feet, with your thumbs at the point where the instep joins the ball of the foot. Be aware of your own feet, your grounding, breathing, and "awareness bubble." Tune in up your partner's body as far as you can go, from feet to head if possible. Then release contact.

Separate your "bubble" from your partner and bring it back around yourself. Then take your hands very definitely off your partner and hold them under running water. Make sure that you both feel completely separate again.

THE ENERGETICS OF ESSENTIAL OILS

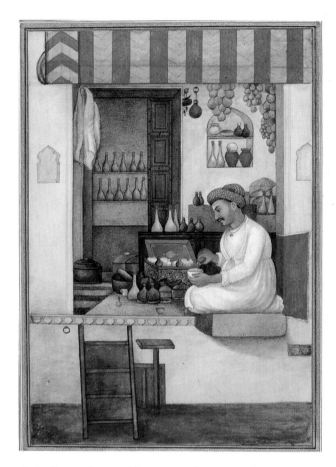

In India, perfumers, like present-day Aromatherapists, are traditionally skilled in selecting the correct scent to suit a mood. This painting by an East India Company artist dates from 1825 and depicts a perfumer in his shop, surrounded by essential oils.

Our sense of smell provides immediate access to our emotions and instincts. According to John Steele, the olfactory epithelium (the small patch of smell receptors that lie at the back of each nostril) is the only part of the nervous system to be directly exposed to the atmosphere —it is on the border between reality and consciousness. It connects through the olfactory bulbs to the limbic system in the brain, where our emotional and instinctual responses originate. Because of this link between scent and awareness, perfume has been used from the earliest civilizations onward to create changes in mood for personal, social, spiritual, or medicinal reasons.

Scent acts on human consciousness in a similar way to music. Both can generate emotional changes, alter mood, summon up images, or recreate memories. The vocabulary of the perfume trade reflects this similarity. Scents consist of base notes, middle notes, and top notes, and the perfumer works from a tall array of shelves, called a "perfume organ." One reason why essential oils can affect human energy so directly is that they resonate at a compatible frequency. This is why essential oils from the living cells of plants and animals are more compatible with human living cells than manufactured scents. Different scent frequencies affect the human energy field in different ways; base notes tend to lower vibrations and so are calming; top notes tend to heighten vibrations and are therefore uplifting; middle notes provide a balance between the two.

Some energetic qualities of a few essential oils are given opposite, but the best way to discover the energy of an oil for yourself is to observe your own responses to it. Inhale the scent of a drop on a tissue and allow the oil to manifest its qualities to you. Try to locate the unique quality of vibration of each oil.

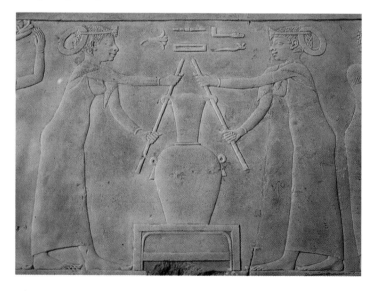

The Egyptians had a great knowledge of aromatics. The flowers in this 4th-century relief are being pressed to extract their essential oils for use in medicines and perfumes.

ESSENTIAL OILS AND THEIR QUALITIES

BASE NOTE SCENTS

Sandalwood

The sweet and earthy smell of sandalwood lulls the mind and is useful in allaying anxiety and mental chatter. In India it is used both as an aphrodisiac and as an incense because of this calming effect. The particular harmonic of its vibration affects both the base chakra and the crown chakra. On the physical level it soothes hot, dry lung and skin conditions and is useful for irritations of the genito-urinary tract.

Frankincense

More uplifting, less earthy in character than sandalwood, frankincense has been found to contain a psychoactive substance that expands consciousness (see *Aromatherapy and the Mind* by Julia Lawless). This accounts for its long history as a meditational aid. It lightens the upper and outer parts of the energy field and increases clarity. On the physical level, like sandalwood, it has affinities with the lungs and skin. It has the effect of deepening the breath.

MIDDLE NOTE SCENTS

Camomile

The best camomiles to use are German camomile or Roman camomile. Both of these oils are similar in action, coming from variants of the herb held sacred first by the Egyptians and later by the Saxons, and used for many centuries as a medicine for body and mind. Camomile relates to the solar plexus and spleen chakras (the spleen has its own chakra, according to many healers), which are linked to security and the polarity between giving and receiving. It calms an active, worried mind, allowing acceptance, and restores the balance between giving and receiving, which is vital if we are to feel security and stability. On the physical level camomile is anti-inflammatory and possesses an affinity with the nervous and digestive systems.

Lavender

Lavender is an excellent "first-aid" remedy and has so many physical uses that its energetic properties are often overlooked. It is useful to combat daily upsets as well as trauma or shock; the oil does this unobtrusively by smoothing and stabilizing the flow of energy throughout the field. The smoothing action cleanses and the stabilizing action comforts, both on the emotional and the physical levels. Its very name comes from the Latin *lavare* "to wash," and the oil's action is to cleanse us of worries and steady us so that we can lead more fulfilling lives.

TOP NOTE SCENTS

Bergamot

Bergamot is a joyous oil, light and delicate with a sparkle and a shimmer in its fragrance. Its carefree quality can loosen the grip of depression associated with bitterness or resentment. It seems to work on the borders of the energy field when they are rigid and contracted, restoring a natural openness and pulsation to the field. On the physical level it restores the natural rhythm of the digestive system and can help with hormonal disruption. However, be careful not to use it on skin that will be exposed to the Sun, as a damaging chemical change can take place. (A version of bergamot that is free of the substances that cause this change is now available.)

Rosemary

Rosemary is well known for its effect as a cephalic, or brain, tonic. The scent initially delivers a powerful "wake-up" jolt and then provides sweet and reliable support for the brain. The senses become more alert and the energy field vibrates at a higher frequency. Rosemary is also good for sluggish livers and aching joints. It should not be used if you are pregnant, breastfeeding, or feverish. It is also not suitable for children aged under two, cases of epilepsy, or high blood pressure.

USING ESSENTIAL OILS

Essential oils for massage should always be diluted in a carrier oil, such as sweet almond or olive oil. Mix the two oils at a ratio of five drops of essential oil to 4 teaspoons (20 ml) of carrier oil and keep the blend in a plastic flip-top bottle. Essential oils can be used in other ways beside massage, such as in baths, inhalations, and compresses. You can perfume a room with a burner or diffuser, or simply inhale a few drops on a tissue.

AN AROMATHERAPY FACE MASSAGE

The mood-altering properties of fragrance can be used most effectively in a face massage. Not only can the essential oils be smelt most strongly here, but the face massage in itself also has a powerfully relaxing and uplifting effect. Research has shown that there is mutual feedback between the brain and the muscles of facial expression. In other words, a frown will make you feel more cross, a smile will make you feel happier. Removing tension from the face muscles therefore helps to soothe the mind. The Zen Shiatsu Master Masunaga told his students that face Shiatsu was good for the soul, and so it feels in practice.

When preparing to give a face massage, make sure that your partner is comfortable and warm, with his or her head at the foot of a bed. (Remember to protect the bed-clothes with a towel.) If you have long hair, tie it back, and move your partner's hair out of the way. It is hard to prevent a little oil from getting on the hair and even harder to do a good massage when you are worrying about it, so make sure that your partner knows this. If you are massaging a man, it will be better for both of you if his face is not stubbly.

Mix up your oil, using a low dilution of five drops of essential oil for about every 4 teaspoons (20 ml) of carrier oil and have it handy in a squeezy bottle. Kneel behind your partner, or sit on a low stool, depending on the height of the bed.

Before beginning the massage, "float" your hands down to your partner's chest and tune in to your own breathing. Become aware of your energy field and extend it to surround your partner; create your "awareness bubble." Oil the entire surface of your partner's upper chest and shoulders, neck, and face with long, sweeping strokes. Start with effleurage to the neck and shoulders as described on page 84.

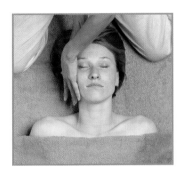 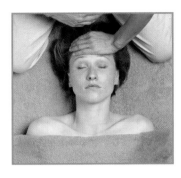 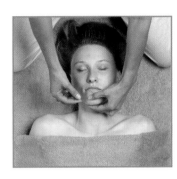 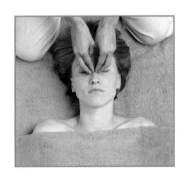

1 *Mould your relaxed hands to your partner's face and stroke, hand over hand, up one cheek from jaw to temple. Use long strokes upward and outward, covering the cheek several times and working slowly and rhythmically. Then, without stopping your rhythm, repeat on the other cheek.*

2 *Keeping the same rhythm and movement, stroke up your partner's forehead from eyebrow to hairline. Move to the center of the forehead and do some long strokes from the bridge of the nose to the hairline. Imagine ironing away tension from the forehead muscles.*

3 *With your fingertips under your partner's chin and your thumb in the groove below the lower lip, slide across his or her chin, first with one hand, then with the other. The hands should travel in opposite directions. Squeeze the flesh of the chin between fingers and thumbs and then release.*

4 *Relax your hands and, with the pads of your fingertips, make tiny circular movements from the center of the lower lip outward and around the lips. Continue up both sides of the nose to the bridge. Do not press too hard, but imagine you are penetrating below the surface to clear the nasal passages.*

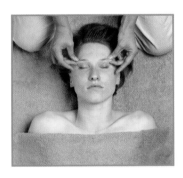 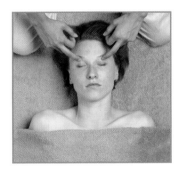 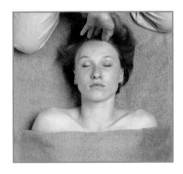

5 *Take the inner ends of your partner's eyebrows between the middle finger and thumb of each hand. Gently pinch and release along the whole eyebrow, sliding your finger along as you go.*

6 *Using your middle fingers, stroke gently from the inner corners of your partner's eyes along the edges of the socket to the outer corners. Return beneath the eyes toward the nose, making very gentle, tiny circular movements. Keep your "awareness bubble" big. Repeat once more.*

7 *Turn your hands so that the palms are facing away from you. Place your fingertips at your partner's hairline and gently rake his or her scalp. Your fingers should be close enough together to pull the hair roots slightly away from the scalp as you repeatedly run your hands through the hair. Cover as much of the scalp as you can reach, and continue for as long as you like; your partner will be floating!*

INTRODUCING REFLEXOLOGY

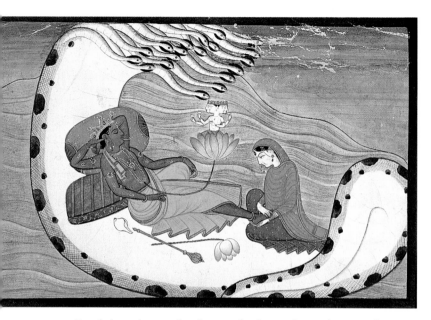

People have known for thousands of years how relaxing a foot massage can be. This 19th-century Indian miniature depicts the Hindu god Vishnu lying on the back of Ananta, the serpent of eternity. His feet are being rubbed by his consort, the goddess Shri.

Reflexology is a therapy that balances your body's energy by accessing it through the feet. It is based on the principle that there are reflexes in the feet (and hands) that relate to every other part of the body. It is said that there are 7,200 nerve endings on the feet from which a complex network allows every part of the body to be accessed. From the feet, nerves run up the legs to the spinal cord from which nerves run to our other limbs, all our internal organs, and our heads. Reflexology gently stimulates parts of the body, helping balance the energy in these parts and allowing the body to heal itself.

Giving such attention to the feet is not a new concept—it has been practiced in many cultures for thousands of years. In the Hamito-Semitic world

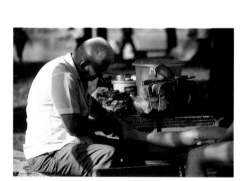

In Thailand, having a foot massage is considered a common and natural way of unwinding. Reflexologists, such as this man in Bangkok, can be seen working on beaches and in parks.

from about 200 B.C.E. to about C.E. 1,900 when a man arrived at a house after a long journey on foot, a good host would wash his feet and massage them in scented oil. At Saqqara in Egypt, wall paintings in the tomb of a very influential physician called Ankhmahor, dated early 6th Dynasty (around 2,330 B.C.E.), include one of a man massaging the foot of a patient. Another shows a patient being given a hand massage.

Clinical studies of how certain areas of the body relate to other parts began in the 1890s with Sir Henry Head, a neurologist in London, England. He discovered that specific areas of skin became sensitive to pressure when an organ was diseased, and realized that these areas and organs were connected by nerves. The field was further explored by Dr William Fitzgerald, an ear, nose, and throat specialist in Connecticut, who found that if he applied constant pressure to parts of the fingers he could induce local anaesthesia elsewhere, and so carry out minor operations without causing pain. Fitzgerald divided the body into ten "zones." By applying pressure or massage to these zones he found he could relieve pain to other areas within the same zone. He published his theories in 1917 in a book, *Zone Therapy*, written with Dr Edwin Bowers. Its concepts were developed by Eunice Ingham (1879–1974), who through testing was able to produce the map of the feet and related zones used by modern Reflexologists.

Energy blockages are caused by stress, sluggish blood circulation, and lack of exercise, all of which promote the accumulation of toxins in the body tissues. In a healthy body these toxins would be eliminated through the urinary system. If they stay in the body, however, they can form crystals that, due to the effect of gravity, often gather under the skin of the feet. A Reflexologist can feel in which parts of the foot the crystals are gathered; the reflexes in these areas correspond to a diseased parts of the body. These areas will therefore often be extremely painful to the recipient of Reflexology when pressure is applied.

Once the painful reflexes and crystals are located, the therapist will massage the area and break up the crystals. This improves the supply of blood and energy to the corresponding part of the body. The toxins are released into the blood stream and flushed out of the system through the kidneys. It is very important to drink 1 pint (50 cl) of water straight after treatment and to carry on drinking extra water over the next 48 hours, and to rest and allow the body to complete its healing. Side effects while the toxins are being expelled may include headaches, pimples, and increased urinary or digestive elimination.

Reflexology is a powerful treatment and should be carried out only by a professional. It is unsuitable for those with thrombosis, unstable pregnancy, or active plantar's warts. If you are suffering from any other illness, you should first obtain permission from your doctor.

REFLEXOLOGY CHARTS

Reflexologists still use charts that are based on those produced by Eunice Ingham. These map out the body on the soles of the feet, with the head reflexes in the big toes, the spine running down the inside edge of both feet, and the shoulders on the outside of the feet, just below the little toes. Organs positioned on the right side of the body, such as the liver, are shown to have corresponding reflexes on the right foot. Organs on the left side of the body, such as the heart, have reflex positions on the left foot. The charts below are simplified versions, showing the reflex points of some of the more important body parts.

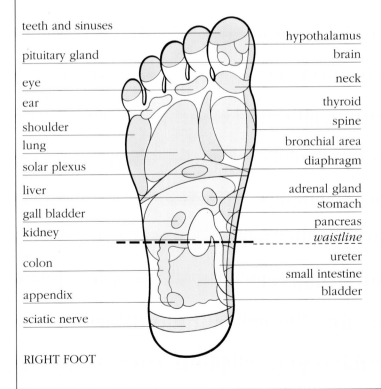

RIGHT FOOT

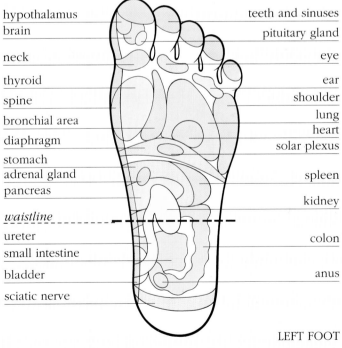

LEFT FOOT

AN ENERGY FOOT MASSAGE

This massage accesses and balances the body's energies through the foot reflexes. If you sit upright in a chair, propping up the foot to be massaged on the opposite knee, you can do many of these exercises to yourself. However, it is more relaxing if a friend applies the massage, and the interaction of two people's energy is very beneficial. Begin on the right foot and then repeat the routine on the left foot.

It is important that you and your partner are comfortable during the massage. You can both sit on chairs with your partner's feet on your lap, or your partner could lie on his or her back on a bed, or with you sitting at his or her feet. Keep eye contact so that you can detect any signs of unease and can communicate with each other.

Your back should be straight, your shoulders relaxed, and your feet flat on the floor. Make sure that your partner's arms are uncrossed, and that you both have removed all watches and jewelry, and loosened any tight clothing. Your hands should be washed and your nails cut short.

A blend of a light oil, such as almond or grapeseed with some peppermint or lemongrass essential oil (see pages 88–9), will help to refresh the feet. A thicker oil, for example jojoba or avocado with drops of frankincense or sandalwood, would be very beneficial if your partner has dry skin. Many Reflexologists find that talcum powder enables a better grip on the foot, allowing a deeper massage, or that using no oil is preferable. Try these alternatives and see which one best suits you and your partner.

GROUNDING

Grounding connects both your and your partner's energies to the Earth. It allows negative energy to flow from your bodies into the Earth and draws positive healing energy into you both from the Earth. Grounding is therefore used to stabilize the energies of both you and your partner. It also helps to calm and focus the mind, and should be done before and after every foot massage.

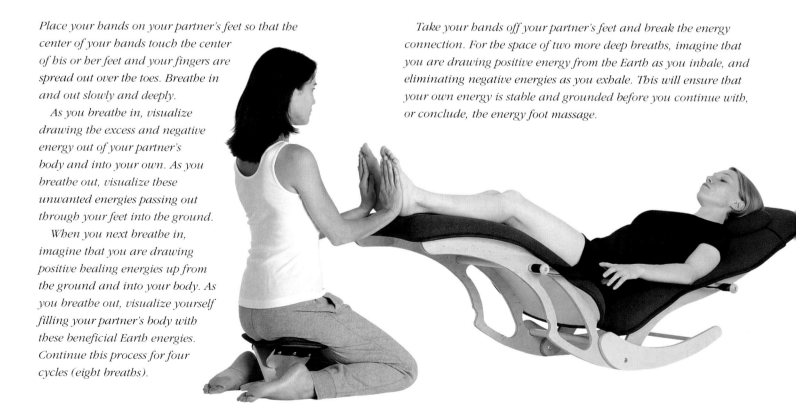

Place your hands on your partner's feet so that the center of your hands touch the center of his or her feet and your fingers are spread out over the toes. Breathe in and out slowly and deeply.

As you breathe in, visualize drawing the excess and negative energy out of your partner's body and into your own. As you breathe out, visualize these unwanted energies passing out through your feet into the ground.

When you next breathe in, imagine that you are drawing positive healing energies up from the ground and into your body. As you breathe out, visualize yourself filling your partner's body with these beneficial Earth energies. Continue this process for four cycles (eight breaths).

Take your hands off your partner's feet and break the energy connection. For the space of two more deep breaths, imagine that you are drawing positive energy from the Earth as you inhale, and eliminating negative energies as you exhale. This will ensure that your own energy is stable and grounded before you continue with, or conclude, the energy foot massage.

SOLAR PLEXUS BREATHING

The solar plexus is a network of nerves that supply the abdominal organs. Pressing the solar plexus reflex can release tension in your partner's diaphragm. In so doing, it may also encourage deep breathing, induce relaxation, and relieve stress and nervousness. This technique also connects the breathing patterns of you and your partner so that your energies can work in harmony.

Place your hands gently on the outside of your partner's feet. Press your thumbs into the center of the sole, in line with the middle toe and just below where the arch meets the ball of the foot. There is a slight dip here—the solar plexus reflex.

Ask your partner to breathe in deeply and to hold his or her breath for ten seconds. As your partner does so, gently press in with your thumbs. As he or she breathes out very slowly, release the pressure and use your fingers to pull the feet gently toward you. Repeat this breathing and pressing exercise six more times.

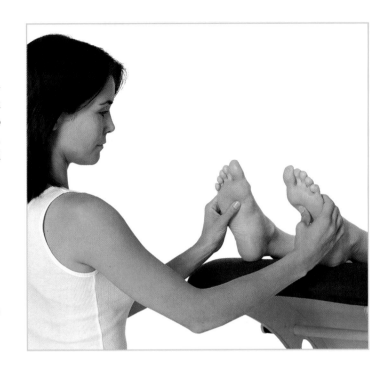

RELAXING THE BODY

Moving thumb over thumb up the sole helps to relax the arches of the feet and remove energy blockages in reflexes of the internal organs, especially the digestive system, lungs, and heart. Rubbing assists in releasing tension and excess energies in the feet, ankles, and calves; it also unlocks tension in the spine, hip, and shoulder girdles. Ankle rotation helps to loosen up and remove energy blockages in the ankle area; in so doing it relaxes the reflexes of the pelvic girdle, colon, and reproductive system.

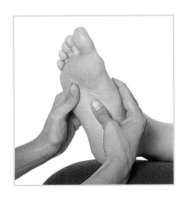

1 Hold the foot gently with the fingers of both hands. With the pads of each thumb in turn, firmly stroke upward on the sole of the foot and outward over the ball toward the base of the toes. Repeat this action until the whole sole of the foot is covered.

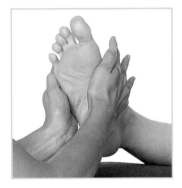

2 Keep your fingers together and place your hands one each side of the foot. Move one hand forward and the other back toward you, twisting the foot gently. Twist briskly in this way for a few minutes, moving both hands up and down the foot, loosening it up all over.

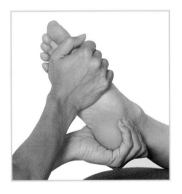

3 Hold your partner's ankle in your left hand and the ball of his or her foot in your right hand. Move the ball of the foot in horizontal circular movements clockwise and then counterclockwise. As it loosens up, you may find that you can move it gently in larger circles.

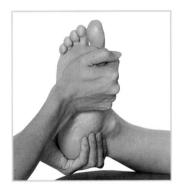

4 Using your right hand, push the ball of the foot away from you, toward your partner's leg, to stretch the tendons in the arch of the foot gently. (When repeating stages 3 and 4 on the left foot, make sure that you also swap the grips of your hands.)

RELIEVING HEADACHES AND TENSION

By releasing tension in the big toes through rotation, stress is also reduced in the neck and upper spine reflexes, allowing energy to flow freely between head and body. The caterpillar walk on the big toe is used to treat all reflexes of the head and neck, promoting endocrine balance, relieving headaches, migraine, hormone imbalances, and neck tension. The benefit of thumb over thumb up the spine is that it massages the spine reflex. It helps energy to flow through the back, relaxing the nerves and muscles that run between the spine, limbs, and organs. Twisting the foot loosens the spine, making the latter more supple to facilitate energy flow.

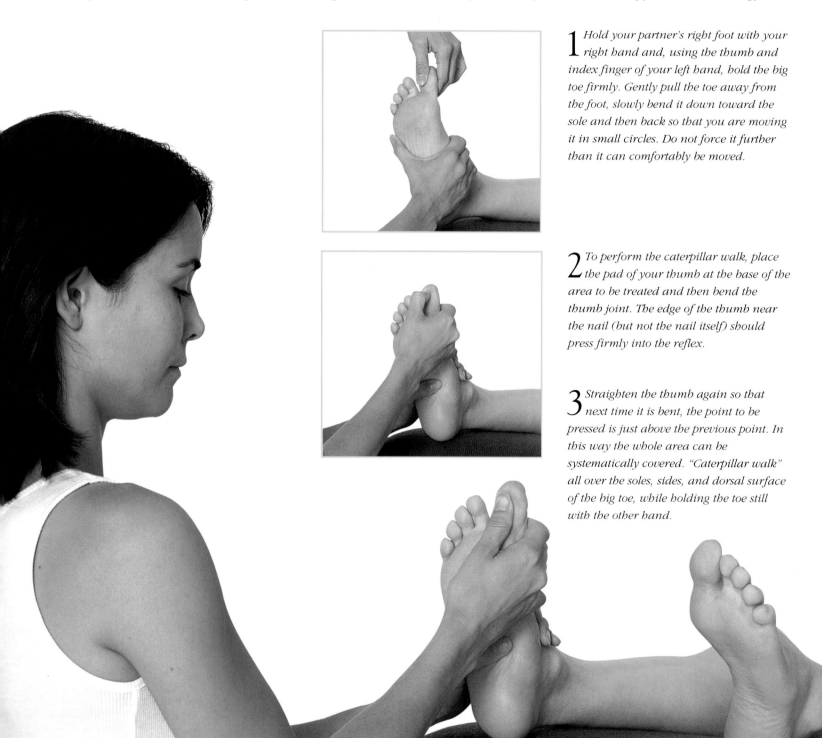

1 *Hold your partner's right foot with your right hand and, using the thumb and index finger of your left hand, hold the big toe firmly. Gently pull the toe away from the foot, slowly bend it down toward the sole and then back so that you are moving it in small circles. Do not force it further than it can comfortably be moved.*

2 *To perform the caterpillar walk, place the pad of your thumb at the base of the area to be treated and then bend the thumb joint. The edge of the thumb near the nail (but not the nail itself) should press firmly into the reflex.*

3 *Straighten the thumb again so that next time it is bent, the point to be pressed is just above the previous point. In this way the whole area can be systematically covered. "Caterpillar walk" all over the soles, sides, and dorsal surface of the big toe, while holding the toe still with the other hand.*

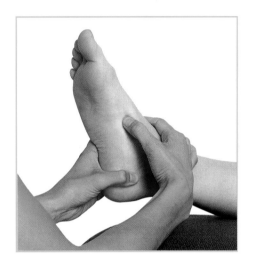

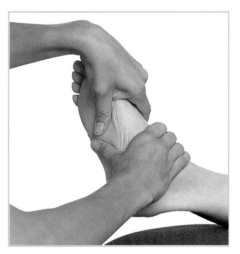

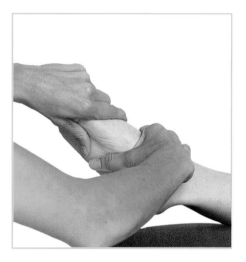

4 *Gently place the fingers of your left hand on the sole and the fingers of your right hand on the dorsal surface of your partner's foot. Using each thumb in turn, apply deep stroking movements up the line of bones that runs along the inside of the foot. Be aware of spine reflexes— such as the waist at the foot's arch, the shoulders at the curve of the ball of the foot, the neck at the base of the big toe— as you massage these areas.*

Then massage up the foot between the line of bones and the sole (this area contains the reflexes for the nerves and muscles beside the spine).

5 *Hold your partner's foot firmly, with the fingers of both hands on the dorsal surface of the foot and the thumbs on the plantar surface or sole. Now gently, and at the same time, move your hands in opposite directions, as if you are wringing the foot out. Keep eye contact with your partner to ensure you do not go too far.*

6 *Slowly move both hands up the foot while continuing this twisting action, until you have covered all of the spinal reflexes. Your partner should not feel a burning sensation on the skin. If he or she does, then you are allowing your hands to slip—applying some talcum powder to improve your hands' grip should help.*

CONCLUSION

To remove excess energy from the body that may have built up during the massage, first massage the big toe. Then, with your thumb and index finger, gently pinch the end of the toe. Slowly pull your finger and thumb away from the toe, as if you were drawing a thread, until you are 1 ft (30 cm) away. Finally, flick your hand as if shaking the energy away. Imagine that you are throwing away this excess energy into the air to be used beneficially elsewhere. Repeat this process with the other toes.

Now repeat the solar plexus breathing and grounding exercises (see pages 94–5). Tell your partner to drink plenty of water and if possible to relax for the rest of the day.

TIBETAN ENERGY MASSAGE

The Tibetan medical system is based on four ancient texts known as the *Gyushi* (*rGyud-bzhi*) or *Four Tantras*. These texts date back to the 8th century C.E. and are said to be an authentic account of the teachings of the Buddha when he took on the form of the Medicine Buddha. The texts not only contain some ideas present in earlier Indian and Chinese texts but also material unique to Tibetan medicine.

The *Four Tantras* consist of the *Root Tantra*, the *Explanatory Tantra*, the *Instructional Tantra,* and the *Subsequent Tantra.* The *Root Tantra* gives a summary of how the various branches of Tibetan medicine are related to each other. As its name suggests, the *Explanatory Tantra* gives a clear and detailed account of the make-up of the human body, from pre-conception to death. It also covers the effects, diagnosis, and treatment of disease.

The most extensive of the *Four Tantras* is the *Instructional Tantra*, which profiles every disease known at the time and suggests methods of diagnosis

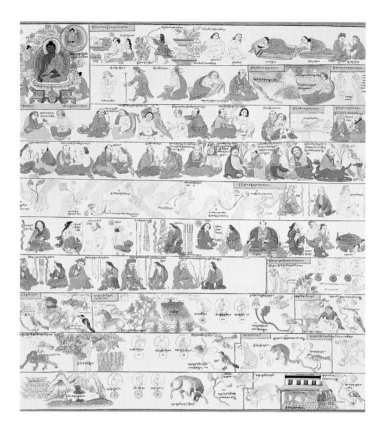

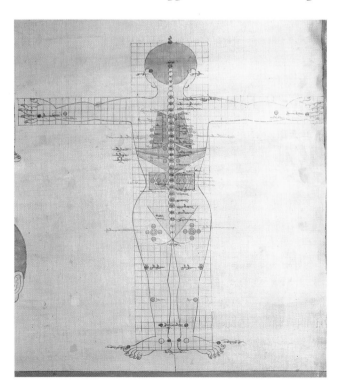

The similarities between Tibetan medicine and Ayurveda are revealed in this painting (above). It describes how the human pulse varies with lifestyle, time, place, and season.

The Tibetan energy system is shown in this back view of a standing man (left) from an 18th-century commentary on the Four Tantras.

and treatment. The *Subsequent Tantra* is a more practical guide to diagnosis and therapy.

The Tibetan medical system views the body as a complex network of both physical and subtle energy channels. The physical channels carry blood, fluids, and nutrients, while the subtle channels carry life force and vitality. There are said to be 72,000 such channels in the body, and these interconnect at five major energy centers (known as chakras or *tsa'khor*) that act as the interface between physical and subtle energy, both receiving and transmitting energy. This concept has many similarities with the Indian *nadi* system of subtle energy channels that can be accessed when performing many of the *asanas* (postures) and *pranayama* (breathing exercises) of Hatha Yoga (see pages 44–5).

In the Tibetan view of energy, there are 24 channels radiating from each energy center, and all of these have vital energy points along them, similar to the acupoints of Traditional Chinese Medicine (see page 18). By pressing these points Tibetan physicians are able to gain information about a patient's energy levels and can locate any blockages. The most expert physicians can diagnose a condition simply by taking the patient's pulse.

Massaging the energy points can promote and balance the flow of energy in the body. In Tibetan medicine there is a system of energetic exercises known as Kum Nye (pronounced "koom neeay"). These exercises are referred to briefly in the *Four Tantras* but have largely been handed down by word of mouth. Although much of the original Kum Nye system has been lost, some exercises have been recorded and adapted to modern life. These exercises aim to integrate body, mind, and spirit by activating the subtle energy system and promoting the flow of energy within both the subtle and the physical channels of the body. Most of the exercises are stationary, or require just small movements or gentle massage of the energy points in the body. The focus is internal rather than external, as awareness of the body is increased and relaxation is deepened in order to expand the range of sensation and depth of feeling.

Tibetan abdominal massage helps to develop stamina, courage, and confidence; it also improves digestion.

TIBETAN ABDOMINAL MASSAGE

This exercise stimulates energetic flow in the abdomen, massages the abdominal organs, and improves digestion. The chest is also opened and blocked feelings may come to the surface, thereby purifying and cleansing the body. The subtle energy center in the abdomen is said to be the seat of vitality in the body, so this exercise also increases vitality and self-confidence.

1 *Lie on the floor with your knees bent and your abdomen relaxed. Place your left palm over the breastbone and your right palm just below your navel. Close your eyes and let your breathing become deep and relaxed.*

2 *Rotate your right palm slowly around the abdomen in a clockwise direction, seven times. Then bring your palm to rest just below the navel. Take deep, relaxed breaths while holding the palms stationary and focusing on the sensations within.*

3 *Reverse the palms for a moment, bringing the energy from the abdominal center to the heart, and vice versa. Observe the changing sensations.*

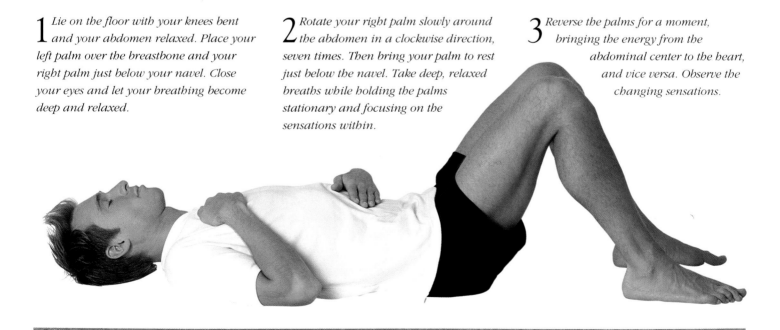

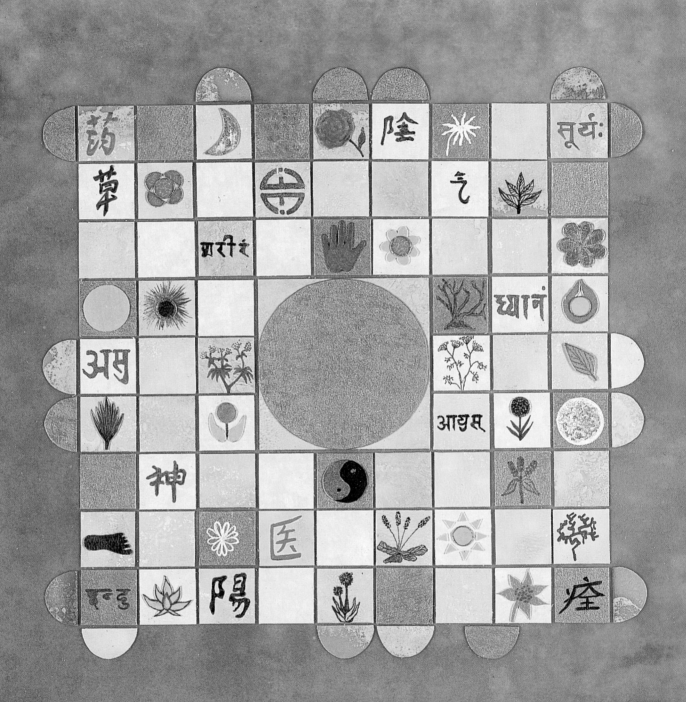

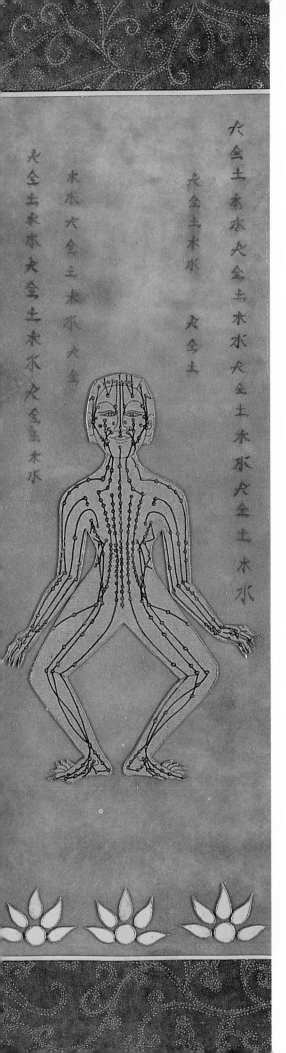

ENERGY, HEALING, AND HARMONY

Today a whole range of therapies, from the ancient to those developed more recently, fall into the new category of "Energy Medicine." Based on the principle that we all have a subtle energy system that needs as much care as our physical bodies, they are gaining in popularity and availability. Such therapies are preventative and corrective and include Acupressure, Acupuncture, Ayurvedic Medicine, Homeopathy, Kinesiology, Polarity Therapy, and Spiritual Healing.

All these systems are based on the premise that ill-health can be detected in the energy system before manifesting in the body, and use different methods of diagnosis or assessment. This chapter offers advice on how to maintain general health, drawing on the principles of Energy Medicine.

HOLISTIC THERAPIES

Holistic therapists see human beings in terms of their bodies, minds, emotions, and spirits. They believe that all these components interact with and affect each other, and that they all need to be in harmony for complete health and well-being. Many holistic therapies either originated in the East (these include Acupuncture, Acupressure, and Ayurveda), or were developed in the West from Eastern concepts of the body's energy. Examples from the latter group include Kinesiology and Polarity Therapy.

When examining a patient, a good holistic therapist will not just look at symptoms but will question the causes. This might involve considering the patient's lifestyle, diet, relationships, and occupation. Recurrent headaches, for example, could be triggered by physical, nutritional, environmental, or emotional stress, and it may be necessary to treat every aspect of the person to bring about a lasting cure.

Both mental and emotional attitudes are included in the whole picture that a holistic therapist tries to develop. Depression and stress create blocks in the energy field and can give rise to physical symptoms: in the holistic vision, both the symptoms and the stress need to be addressed. Conversely, an apparently emotional problem may have physical causes—a sensitivity or allergy to certain foods, or even an unbalanced diet, can affect brain and body chemistry, leading to depression. This in turn affects the energy system. Similarly, lack of exercise can lead to a lack of natural endorphins in the body, which can result in mental and physical sluggishness.

Some holistic therapists—such as colonic hydrotherapists (who practice colonic irrigation), Ayurvedic doctors, some massage therapists, and Aromatherapists—maintain that our bodies are poisoned by the toxins contained in the food that we eat and the polluted atmosphere that

This Chinese bronze Acupuncture figure has holes that relate to the acupoints in the body. It would have been used to show students where to place the needles.

we breathe. "Toxic" products include coffee, tea, sugar, and processed foods, as well as nicotine and alcohol. Many therapists say that all of these substances should be avoided during a detoxification program, which offers the first step toward well-being.

Practitioners of "energy medicine" believe that many problems begin in the energy field at an early stage, even at birth, and are compounded by stresses later in life. A childhood trauma, for example, may weaken the heart center; physically this could be reflected in round shoulders and a narrow chest, creating respiratory problems such as asthma. This in turn can be exacerbated by air pollution and diet. Treatment in such a case would need to address the patient's breathing, posture, and lifestyle, but might also require counseling to heal the original trauma.

Holistic therapists have various ways of measuring a patient's energy flow and identifying blockages or imbalances. Acupuncturists and Ayurvedic practitioners gauge the energy of the meridians through the pulses. Kinesiologists test muscles in relation to the energy system. Healers may sense or even see problems latent in the energy field. Weaknesses or imbalances in the chakras can be sensed by the hand of a skilled practitioner. Alternatively, they can be revealed by dowsing with a pendulum. All these methods have the advantage that, if used early on, they can prevent illness.

Using techniques such as Kinesiology to assess a person's physical and energy states, holistic practitioners can often trace the root causes of their problems. They frequently involve patients in their own healing process and support them in making positive changes in their attitudes and lifestyles.

ACUPUNCTURE

Thousands of years ago the Chinese recognized that the body's essential energy (Qi) flows through the body via channels now called meridians, which carry energy to and from the body's glands and organs. Acupuncture aims to maintain good physical and emotional health by encouraging Qi to flow harmoniously. Along each meridian lie many acupoints, through which low energy can be boosted or excess energy reduced, by inserting needles that are almost as fine as a hair.

Traditional Acupuncturists check the state of the meridians through the strength and quality of the pulses (six on each wrist, see page 18), before giving the appropriate treatment. Some also advise on diet or prescribe herbal medicine.

The acupoints treated will be chosen according to the practitioner's diagnosis and may therefore vary from session to session as the patient's condition improves. Acupuncture needles are usually made of stainless steel. When they are inserted there should be little or no pain, although some people find it uncomfortable and others feel a strange, tingling sensation within the limb. This should be encouraged as it is said to be the Qi arriving at the needle.

Needles are usually inserted to a depth of around ½ inch (1cm), but they can go as deep as 4 inches (12 cm), depending on which part of the body the Acupuncturist is treating. Sometimes the needles are manipulated between the practitioner's first finger and thumb in order to increase their effect. Treatments usually last between 20 and 30 minutes, although they can be longer.

Acupuncturists sometimes also use other traditional Chinese medicine therapies, such as Moxibustion and Cupping. Derived from the Japanese word *mogusa*, meaning "burning herb," the aim of Moxibustion is to warm the Qi traveling around the body. It is often used to drive out infections, to increase the energy of a specific point, or to relieve pain. During a session, the practitioner places a small cone of the dried or shredded leaves of a herb, usually common mugwort, over an acupoint, either at the end of a needle or close to the skin. This is repeated several times on the same point. Some practitioners use a moxa box to apply heat over a larger area of the body. This is particularly useful when treating dull, non-specific pain such as backache or period pain.

Cupping is also used to warm the blood and Qi flowing through the body. A lighted piece of cotton wool is placed in

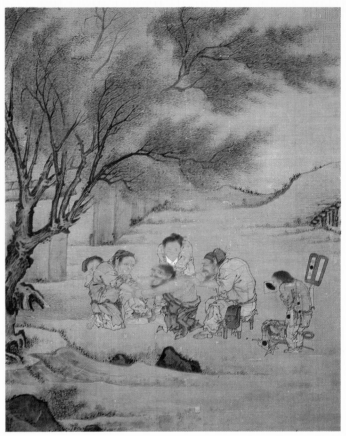

A painting by Li Tang, dating from the Song Dynasty (C.E. 906–1279). It depicts a country doctor applying Moxibustion to a patient's back. This involves either burning herbs near to the skin, or attaching the herbs to an inserted Acupuncture needle.

either a glass or, traditionally, a bamboo cup for a few minutes. Withdrawing the cotton wool creates a vacuum in the cup, so that the vessel remains in place when it is placed strategically on the skin. The cup is left on the body for a few more minutes, where it draws the blood to the surface. This may result in bruising, which should quickly fade.

Because the purpose of Acupuncture is to rebalance the Qi flowing through your meridians, it is possible that after being treated you will feel a difference in your energy levels. Initially, you may feel elated or tired. These feelings should become less strong with treatment as your energy flow is regulated. It is advisable to rest and avoid stimulants after a treatment.

ACUPRESSURE

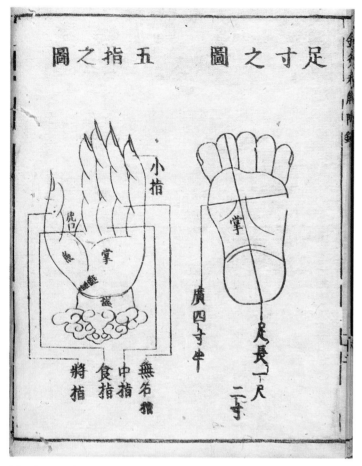

This late 17th-century illustration shows acupoints in the hand and foot. It is a rare example of a Japanese commentary on a Chinese medical text that was first printed in 1341.

The healing art of Acupressure dates back thousands of years and has its roots in Oriental medicine. It involves the application of fingertip pressure to vital energy points, known as acupoints, on the body in order to stimulate the flow of energy and promote health. In Traditional Chinese Medicine there are around 365 acupoints along the 12 main meridians (see pages 18–19) of the body. Some are major points with powerful effects on the body while others are less strong. The system can be compared to a rail network in which the meridians are the railway lines, the major acupoints the main terminals, and the minor acupoints the small local stations.

Pressure may be applied to the acupoint with the fingertips (most usually the index or middle fingers), the thumbs, or with tools such as small pointed wooden pressure sticks or specially designed small metal rollers.

First the point has to be located correctly through body measurement, anatomical placement, and touch. Next, gentle pressure is applied either perpendicularly into the skin or in the direction of energy flow in the meridian according to Oriental medical principles. The pressure may be maintained evenly or by means of small rotations. It is then gently released.

Acupressure should never be painful but sensations of dullness or tingling are not uncommon. There should be a definite sense of pressure, but it should be released if it becomes painful. Most points are bilateral, so pressure has to be applied on both sides of the body. The exceptions are points on meridians that only have one pathway such as those coursing the midline on the front and back of the body. Breathing is crucial during Acupressure because it helps to stimulate the flow of energy. It should always be even and relaxed. Visualization of improved energetic flow, or of the relief of the current symptom, can also be helpful.

The application of pressure to the point stimulates and regulates the flow of vital energy in the body. It is also said to trigger natural homeostatic mechanisms, and in this way the same point can be used for either an excess or a deficiency condition in the body.

Acupressure can easily be practiced by anyone. No special equipment or skills are required—simply practice in locating the points and applying pressure correctly. It can be used to boost vitality, promote healing, and relieve common ailments. The only contraindications for Acupressure are pregnancy (where care has to be taken to avoid the points that promote labor) and intoxication (it should never be carried out when someone is under the influence of alcohol or non-medicinal drugs). Care must also be taken to apply only very light pressure in the case of babies and children, the elderly, or the frail.

ACUPRESSURE POINTS

Pressing a combination of points can be useful in promoting and regulating energy flow in the body. Begin by rubbing your palms to warm your hands and stretching out each finger. Take care to locate the points correctly, and then apply pressure in an even and sustained way. Keep your body relaxed and breathe evenly. A few minutes' practice twice a day is more effective than longer, but less regular periods of practice. Usually between 30 and 60 seconds' stimulation to a point is sufficient: otherwise it may become sore.

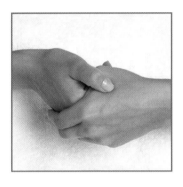

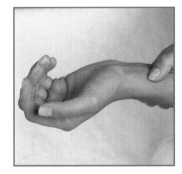

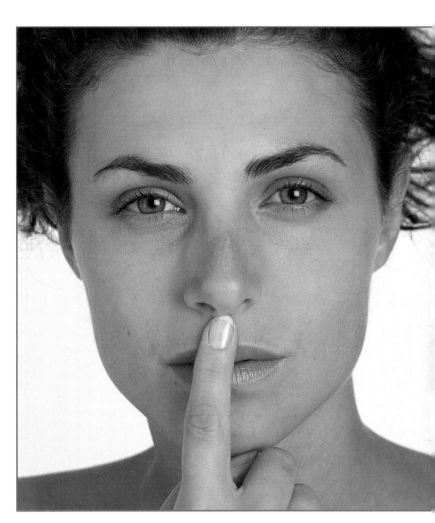

1 Located in the middle of the angle between the thumb and index finger, Large Intestine 4 is a potent point. It stimulates the energy flow in the upper body, clears the skin, improves the complexion, stimulates mental awareness, and aids digestive function.

Support beneath the web of your left thumb and index finger with the fingers of your right hand, and apply pressure straight down using your right thumb. Repeat, applying pressure to your right hand. This acupoint should not be stimulated during pregnancy.

2 Located on the inside of the wrist in line with the thumb, Lung 7 is in the hollow behind the wrist bone about two fingers' width from the wrist crease. This acupoint is used to strengthen the lungs and respiratory function, to increase overall vitality and to prevent or ease breathing problems, such as bronchitis or asthma.

Support below your left wrist with the fingers of your right hand, and apply pressure with your right thumb angled down toward the hand. Repeat on your right wrist.

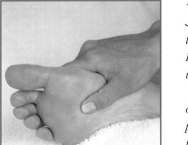

3 Located just below the ball of the foot, in the hollow a third of the way along the sole, Kidney 1 is used to boost vitality and relieve fatigue.

Sit with your right foot held on your left knee, and apply pressure with your right thumb. Now repeat the process on your left foot.

4 Located in the groove above the upper lip, just below the nose, Governor Vessel 26 is a very useful acupoint. When it is pressed, its many benefits include improved mental alertness, concentration, and memory. It can also be used when applying First Aid, to relieve feelings of faintness and has even been known to help restore consciousness.

Using either your left or right hand, gently apply pressure with the tip of your index finger or the edge of your fingernail. Pressure should be perpendicular into the groove.

KINESIOLOGY

Kinesiology is a general term to describe the various holistic therapies that combine manual muscle testing with the principles of Traditional Chinese Medicine. The oldest of the therapies, Applied Kinesiology (AK), was founded in 1964 by an American Chiropractor, George Goodheart, who discovered that muscles have energy connections with the meridians (see pages 18–19). Although links had already been established between the subtle energy of the meridians and the functioning of the physical body's organs and glands, Goodheart showed that it was possible to measure the body's energy through muscle testing. This opened up new possibilities for diagnosis and treatment of the physical body by working with subtle energy.

When testing a muscle, the body should be positioned so that the muscle is contracted and as isolated as possible from the other muscles it works with. The practitioner then applies light pressure for a couple of seconds, trying to extend the muscle. If the muscle moves more than 2 inches (5 cm) it is considered weak; if it holds, it is considered strong.

The big muscle in the front of the thigh that helps to raise the leg when walking is called the quadriceps muscle. Kinesiologists teach that this muscle has an energy connection with the small intestine meridian—the small intestine is the part of the body where nutrients are absorbed from food. If this muscle is weak when tested, it might not only result in tiredness when walking but could also indicate poor energy flow to the small intestine meridian and to the small intestine itself. This inadequate flow of energy could result in nutritional deficiencies, which could in turn cause health problems. A Kinesiologist would re-test the muscle to find out what treatment was needed to strengthen it and ultimately to restore energy flow to both the meridian and organ. As a result of strengthening the quadriceps muscle and the energy flow to its meridian, the function of the small intestine would be improved and health restored.

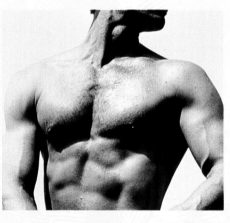

Kinesiologists teach that it is possible to locate energy imbalances in the subtle body through testing the muscles of the physical body.

Other examples can be found in the two large upper chest muscles, known as the pectoralis major clavicular muscles, that assist in movements of the shoulder and arm. These are associated with the stomach meridian and the stomach. If the pectoral muscles are tested and found to be weak, this could indicate that there is a poor flow of energy to the stomach, which in turn could suggest digestive or other physical problems in the present and the future. Most of the surface muscles in the body have similar connections to meridians and organs and can be tested in this way.

Muscle testing can also be used to find out the body's response to foods, thoughts, colors, and treatments. If a strong muscle goes weak when a person is having a particular thought, then that thought is causing stress, which is weakening the system. Similarly, if the muscle weakens when a certain food is tasted, it could indicate an allergy to that food.

Kinesiology aims to balance all aspects of a person—structural, chemical, mental, and emotional—by putting the body in the optimum state for self-healing. Practitioners may suggest a variety of treatments and advice, including exercises to strengthen weak muscles and the flow of energy in their corresponding meridians, changes in diet and the taking of nutritional supplements, and counseling to deal with emotional issues. Kinesiology can be of benefit to people of all ages and states of health. It can be applied in any walk of life and can assist athletes, performers, and people with dyslexia. Its main strength is in prevention, as it aims to create and maintain good health and well-being.

Touch for Health, the lay person's Kinesiology, is a self-help health enhancement training open to everyone. It was developed by American practitioner John Thie in 1973 for non-professional use with family and friends. Touch for Health is not used to diagnose or to treat symptoms, but rather generally to improve and balance the flow of energy through the body. The Kinesiology exercises given in *Your Body's Energy* are taught in Touch for Health workshops throughout the world.

Although Kinesiologists use muscle testing as a means of assessment and to select effective treatments, many of the treatments can be performed safely by yourself, without prior testing. You can release emotional stress and improve your coordination, vision, hearing, and general health. The exercises and treatments are quick and easy to do, taking just a few minutes every day, and can be fitted into a busy life. It is amazing how quickly you can benefit from them. Try them and find out for yourself.

INTEGRATION

We may not be aware of integration explicitly, but we all respond to the effects. If we are well integrated, we function more effectively and feel better.

Our brain has two hemispheres, each of which processes information differently. One side is more involved in the process of logical thinking; the other side is more involved in perceiving patterns, shapes, and rhythms. Because each hemisphere controls the opposite side of the body from the eyes down, we function less efficiently in both mental and physical terms if the hemispheres are badly integrated. Kinesiology offers many exercises to enhance our integration, such as the Cross Crawl (see page 72), Cook's Hook-up (see page 109), and the specific Integration Exercise (see page 73).

We can enjoy a feeling of integration in mind and body by performing the emotional stress release exercise (see page 143), which activates the brain's two hemispheres to bring about emotional balance. This harmonizes the

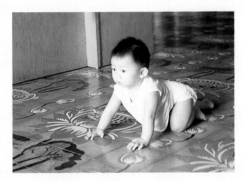

Crawling is an important stage in our physical and mental development. It encourages communication between the two sides of the brain.

emotional centers located in these hemispheres and has a profound effect on the body's physiology as a whole.

In order to feel fully integrated, we also need to have all our senses well tuned and working as an integrated whole. You can improve your vision, for example, by activating certain acupoints. Place one hand over your navel. With the other hand, massage two points just under your collar bone on each side of your breast

bone—about 4 inches (10 cm) apart. As you do this, keep your head straight, but move your eyes very slowly, rotating them all the way round in one direction and then back again. See the difference.

Our ears also play an important part in our overall feeling of balance and integration. They contain a map of our whole body and Auricular Acupuncture specializes in applying needles to the ears alone. We can activate these points and affect our hearing and our whole body by massaging our ears.

To activate the reflexes, turn your head as far as you can all the way to one side, and then the other. Now firmly smooth out the folds in your ears, moving from the top down and from the inside out. Notice the difference. Ear massage is suggested by Kinesiologists to improve hearing; clear tinnitus (a ringing, hissing, or booming sensation in the ears); aid balance; reduce travel sickness; balance bones in the cranium (skull); clear headaches and provide a feeling of clarity and lightness.

POLARITY SWITCHING

Kinesiologists teach that throughout our bodies we have in-built positive (south) and negative (north) poles. The power of these poles can be affected by stress: structural, mental, emotional, chemical, and environmental factors can all contribute to imbalances in our bodies' poles. These in turn cause a breakdown in our bodies' communications and irregularities in energy flow.

By alternating positive and negative charges quickly on a patient's body (polarity switching), Kinesiologists can detect polarity imbalances. Correcting these imbalances involves massaging important acupoints to re-establish communication. If a feeling of disorientation persists, consult a qualified Kinesiologist to discover the root cause.

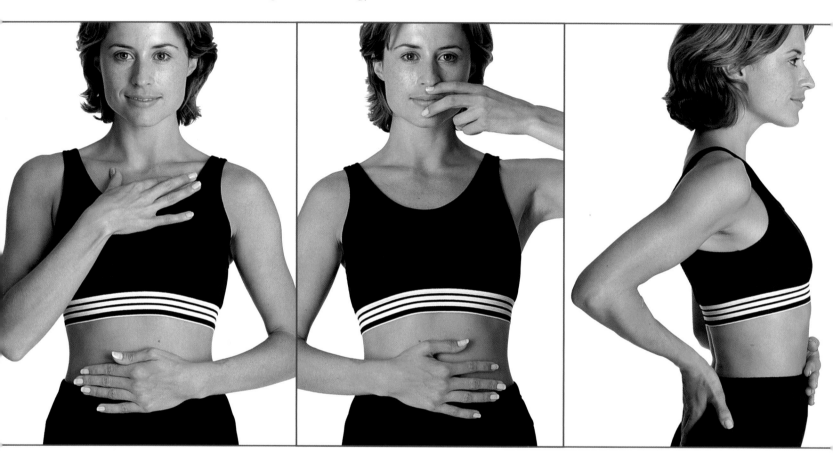

1 Put one hand over your navel. Using the thumb and fingers of the other hand, simultaneously massage two points about 4 inches (10 cm) apart, just below your collar bone on each side of the breastbone. Massage gently for about ten seconds. This helps to balance the energy flow in the Kidney Meridian (see page 19).

2 Keep one hand on your navel and massage two points, one on the upper lip and one on the lower lip, for about ten seconds. The point on the upper lip is on the Governor Vessel (see page 19) and helps to regulate Yang energy. That on the lower lip is on the Conception Vessel, which is used to regulate Yin energy.

3 Still with your hand on your navel, massage the very base of your spine, the coccyx, for about ten seconds. This is another point on the Governor Vessel.

Now repeat the sequence, covering your navel with the opposite hand and using the other hand to massage. To conclude the exercise, breathe deeply and relax.

COOK'S HOOK-UP

Many complementary therapies draw upon the ancient Chinese concepts of Qi and meridian theory (see pages 16–19) to correct energy imbalances and blockages within the body. If the body is under stress or in shock, its reservoirs of energy may be low and the flow of energy in the meridians may be depleted, blocked, or even reversed. Cook's Hook-up is a Kinesiology exercise that involves putting the body into a particular posture to reconnect meridian energy and stimulate a balanced, healthy flow.

This exercise takes only ten minutes to complete and will significantly improve your energy levels, sleep pattern, and ability to deal positively with stress.

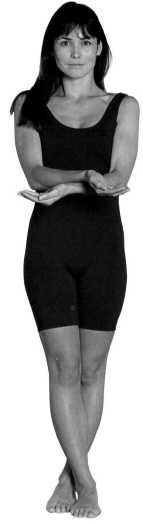

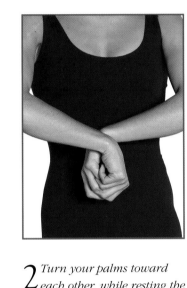

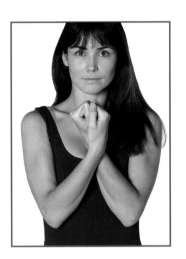

1 Cross your right leg over your left leg and place both feet firmly on the ground. Then cross your right arm over your left arm with your hands palm-upward in front of you. Take time to balance, gather your thoughts, and relax.

2 Turn your palms toward each other, while resting the sides of your hands very lightly on your stomach. Link the fingers together and curl them into the palm of the opposite hand so that they appear to be symmetrical. Hold for 30 seconds, breathing deeply from the abdomen.

3 Turn the fingers upward so that they are in front of the chest. The backs of the hands should now be facing forward. Place your tongue on the roof of your mouth and breathe deeply, visualizing energy flowing easily around your body. Retain this position for one minute.

4 Uncross your arms and legs, and place your feet firmly on the ground. Put your hands together so that only your fingertips touch. Place your tongue on the roof of your mouth and breathe deeply. Hold this position for one minute.

Repeat the sequence, leading with the opposite leg and hand.

HEALING AND THERAPEUTIC TOUCH

Healing through touch or thought may be the oldest form of energy medicine (it was certainly known to the ancient Egyptians and Greeks). It has many names, including "spiritual," "psychic," "etheric," and "hands-on" healing.

Seen for centuries as either miraculous or fraudulent, such healing is now gaining in respectability. Scientific studies have shown that healing energy has beneficial effects on human, plant, and animal cells, showing that it is not dependent on faith or belief. A small but growing number of healers now work with doctors, while some complementary therapists, such as massage therapists and Osteopaths, incorporate healing into their work.

In the 1970s Dolores Krieger, an American professor of nursing, studied the work of healers under scientific conditions. She established that healing has genuine physical effects (such as raising haemoglobin levels in the blood) and also found that most people had the innate ability to heal. Krieger developed a healing system known as Therapeutic Touch; it is taught only to the nursing profession and has spread widely throughout the world.

During a healing session, energy is transmitted from one person to another, usually through the hands. This transmission triggers the receiver's self-healing capacity. Some healers use their own energy ("magnetic healing"), but this can be depleting; most regard themselves as vehicles for a universal energy that can heal at all levels—spiritual, mental, emotional, and physical. These healers can be said to act as transmitters through which energy is transferred. Most healers use only their hands and often work in the energy field without touching the body. Some also use crystals, sound, and color.

Healing can help to boost the immune system and restore depleted energy. Its ability to relieve pain is particularly useful for long-term problems, such as arthritis. Its effects are usually gradual. Miracles are rare, although there have been cases of tumors disappearing. When there is severe deterioration, healing may not have a physical effect but may enable the patient to cope better with his or her illness. Today more and more people are turning to healing for everyday problems and as preventative medicine. Because it works on the energy field, it is useful for emotional and mental problems, helping people to see their difficulties more clearly and to deal with them more effectively.

An electromagnetic or Kirlian photograph showing lines of energy radiating from the surface of the hands. Most healers work with their hands, often in the energy field that surrounds the patient's body. Usually the energy they transmit is not their own but is part of a universal energy that is carried through them.

HEALING, AURAS, AND THE CHAKRA SYSTEM

In the Western model used by healers, energy is not confined to the physical body but surrounds the body in all directions and extends for some distance beyond its surface. This radiant energy is known as the aura. It is invisible to most people, but those who have seen an aura usually it as a large, shimmering oval of light that is arranged into seven differently colored bands or bodies. Each of the bands corresponds to one of the chakras of the Indian system (see pages 44–5).

The individual bands and chakras are believed to relate to several aspects of the body/mind system. Physically they are each connected with the endocrine glands, organs, and spine, and, on the energy level, they are linked with particular emotions and qualities. The state of a person's chakras and aura can therefore reveal a lot of information about him or her to a healer. Many healers use chakras as guidelines for effective healing, helping to energize underactive chakras and calm overactive ones.

When giving healing, healers allow their own higher chakras—particularly the heart and the crown—to open up to universal energy.

The outer band of the aura, known as the cosmic body, emanates from the crown chakra. This in turn is linked to the pineal gland and cerebral cortex in the physical body, and is associated with higher consciousness, spirituality, and inspiration.

The spiritual body emanates from the brow chakra, which is related to the eyes, pituitary gland, and hypothalamus. Its associated qualities are intuition and will.

The causal body emanates from the throat chakra, which is related to the ears, tongue, and throat. Its related qualities are communication, self-expression, as well as the ability to hear and receive.

The heart body emanates from the heart chakra. It is associated with the heart, thymus gland, lungs, and immune system, and feelings of unconditional love.

The mental body emanates from the solar plexus chakra, which is related to the solar plexus, digestive system, and adrenal glands of the physical body, and to self-esteem.

The emotional body emanates from the sacral chakra, which is related to the urogenital system, the intestines, and the lumbar vertebrae. It is linked to sexuality, creativity, and action.

The etheric body emanates from the root or base chakra, which is related to the sacrum, spine, and legs. It is associated with elimination, and with feelings of being grounded, and also to our material survival.

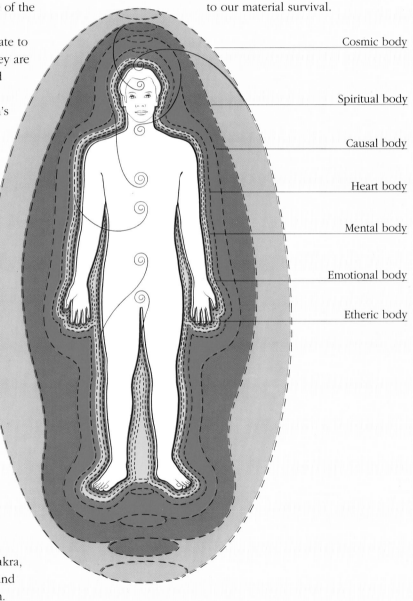

Cosmic body

Spiritual body

Causal body

Heart body

Mental body

Emotional body

Etheric body

GIVING HEALING TO A FRIEND

Anyone who has experienced the energy in their hands, as described on page 25, can learn to transmit it to others. Once achieved, this ability should increase with practice. If you feel you have a gift for healing, there are many professional training courses available.

Before the healing session, perform a Qigong or Yoga exercise to energize your body. Calm your mind by practicing deep breathing for a few minutes. To keep the boundaries between healer and recipient clear, you should protect your energy field: visualize yourself surrounded by a bubble of white or golden light that emits positive energy and shields you from negative energy.

It is important to be well grounded when healing, as you are making yourself available to powerful energies. Remove your shoes and be aware of your feet in contact with the ground. Visualize them growing roots, connecting you with the energy of the Earth. Still standing, mentally open yourself up to the energy of the Sun or a higher wisdom. Imagine a ray of light flowing through your crown center to your heart center, then down your arms to your hands.

If you have a massage table or suitable couch, your friend can lie down. Otherwise, ask him or her to sit in a chair, with legs uncrossed, feet flat on the floor, and his or her shoes removed. Discuss any particular problems that need attention. Then get him or her to relax with two or three deep breaths. If your friend is seated, you can work on both sides of the body simultaneously. If he or she is lying down, start by working on the back and then ask your friend to turn over to give healing to the front of the body.

Be discreet about where and how you touch, and about what you say. You may sense disruption in your friend's physical or emotional state, but it may not be appropriate to mention it. Do not try to make the other person better; effort is counter-productive. Simply have the mental intention and trust that the energy you are transmitting will bring about harmony where it is needed. Never give healing if you are under par yourself.

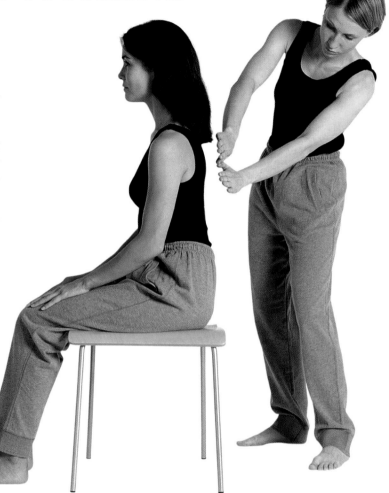

1 *Begin by running your hands down your friend's back, about 1 inch (2.5 cm) in front of the spine. Notice any areas of heat, cold, or tingling. These may indicate an energy block, and possibly physical pain or tension.*

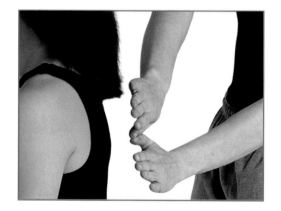

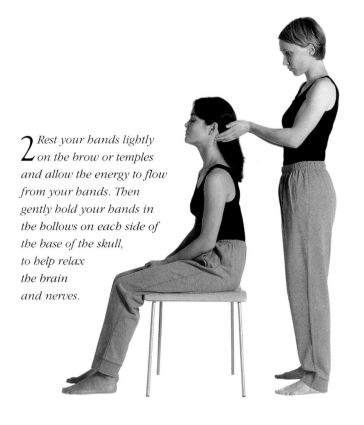

2 *Rest your hands lightly on the brow or temples and allow the energy to flow from your hands. Then gently hold your hands in the hollows on each side of the base of the skull, to help relax the brain and nerves.*

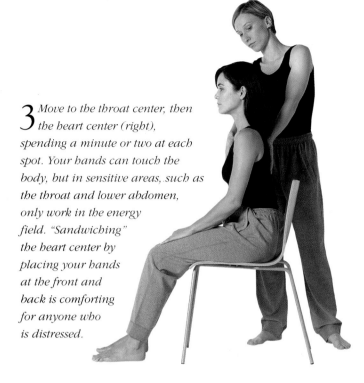

3 *Move to the throat center, then the heart center (right), spending a minute or two at each spot. Your hands can touch the body, but in sensitive areas, such as the throat and lower abdomen, only work in the energy field. "Sandwiching" the heart center by placing your hands at the front and back is comforting for anyone who is distressed.*

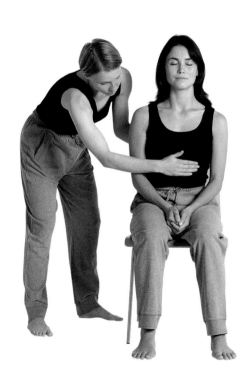

4 *Continue down the body, healing the solar plexus (above), the sacral center, and the base of the spine. With your hands on the solar plexus, ask for feedback; your friend may have felt the energy as heat, coolness, or tingling. Move down to your friend's feet, to ground him or her and help disperse the energy through the body.*

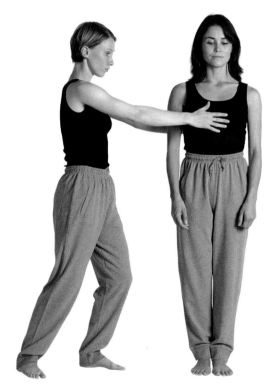

5 *After up to 20 minutes of healing, ask your friend to stand up. "Brush" down his or her energy field with your hands, back and front, sweeping away negative energy that has been released. Both you and your friend should ground yourselves, then wash your hands, imagining the negative energies being flushed away.*

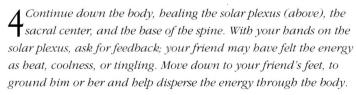

POLARITY THERAPY

Polarity Therapy is a holistic system of healing that encompasses the body, mind, energy system, and spirit. It was developed over 50 years by Dr Randolph Stone (1890–1983), an Austrian-born Naturopath, Chiropractor, and Osteopath. Stone, who also studied Oriental Medicine and spiritual teachings, concluded that energy is the basis of all life.

Drawing on Ayurvedic principles (see pages 118–21) as well as Western concepts, the basic premise of Polarity Therapy is that health and happiness depend on, and can be maintained by, the free flow of energy through the body. Electromagnetic energy flows through positive and negative poles in different parts of the body in a double helix pattern, linking the five lower chakras.

The heart chakra, here depicted as a 12-petaled lotus set around a Star of David and the seed sound YAM, governs inspiration in all its forms.

Each of the chakras can be related to one of the five elements in Chinese and Ayurvedic medicine: ether, air, fire, water, and earth. These in turn affect the chakras' mental and physical attributes. For example, the heart chakra not only relates to the heart but also, through its relationship with the air element, governs the lungs.

CHAKRA	ELEMENT	GOVERNS
Throat	Ether	The emotions, particularly grief
Heart	Air	Conscious desire, mental activity, lungs, nervous system
Solar plexus	Fire	The intellect, anger, eyesight, digestion, and circulation
Sacrum	Water	"Gut" instinct, creativity, procreation, generative and lymphatic systems
Root / Base	Earth	Basic energy, sensations of being grounded, colon, elimination

Energy flows from and to one source in three currents: positive, negative, and neutral. The positive and negative currents flow up and down the body on each side of the spine in a double helix shape. Where they cross each other they create a whirlpool of energy that is a chakra. The neutral current flows along the central column, acting as the body's earth.

According to Dr Stone, all disease arises from disruptions to the flow of energy, which can be reflected in the musculo-skeletal, nervous, circulatory, and digestive systems. Dr Stone also recognized the importance of emotional and mental attitudes that underlie the disease process; negative thoughts and fears create blocks of negative energy. Treatment benefits general health, the digestion, muscular problems, and the emotions. It involves four processes: touch, diet, improvement of mental attitudes, and exercises. Polarity Therapists use therapeutic bodywork, involving gentle touch techniques, to balance the currents and centres of energy. A variety of cleansing diets are suggested to help rid the body of toxins, and a health-building diet appropriate to individual needs is suggested. Treatment with Polarity Therapy also involves counseling to encourage a positive attitude of mind. Progress is supported by a series of simple exercises that help keep the energies free and flowing and that can be related to the chakras and the five elements. Patients are encouraged to take responsibility for their own health.

Dr Stone's system of easy exercises can be practiced by anyone. These consist of gentle stretching and rocking movements, together with some more vigorous exercises using movement and sound to help release blocked energy—sound can be particularly helpful in releasing tensions. Note that it is very important to rest and relax after doing these exercises.

BASIC SQUAT

The basic squat encourages your body's energy to flow and is particularly good for releasing tension in the pelvis. This area is related to the sacral chakra and the element of water.

Lower your body slowly into a squat, with your feet slightly apart. (If necessary, support your heels on a book or cushion.) Circle your body and rock gently to and fro to open up and stretch the body.

WOOD CHOPPER

This exercise is designed to unlock blocked fire energy, which is held in the solar plexus chakra. It is particularly good for releasing pent-up anger, which if stored can both cloud your judgement and lead to indigestion. Make sure that you give an uninhibited shout as you swing down, as this greatly increases the exercise's benefit.

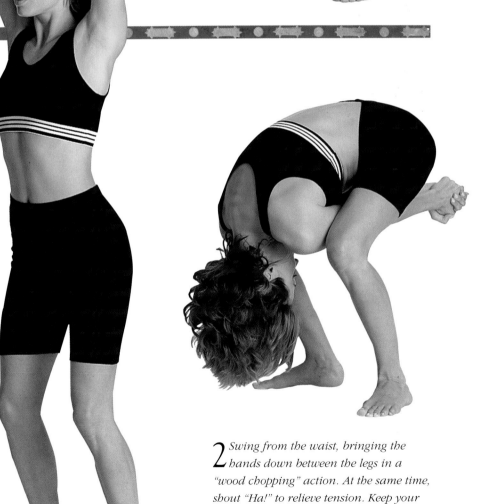

1 *Stand with your feet a hips' width apart. Bend your knees, tilt back your pelvis, and clasp your hands high above your head as if you are holding an axe.*

2 *Swing from the waist, bringing the hands down between the legs in a "wood chopping" action. At the same time, shout "Ha!" to relieve tension. Keep your knees bent throughout the exercise. Repeat as often as comfortable without strain.*

HOMEOPATHY AND FLOWER REMEDIES

An important feature of energy medicine is that treatments work gently, in cooperation with the energy system. In contrast, medical drugs attack symptoms but may have damaging side-effects. A major pioneer in this field was Samuel Hahnemann, a German doctor and chemist who founded Homeopathy in the late 18th century. Disillusioned with the heavy-handed medical practices of the day, he experimented on himself to formulate an entirely new system of medicine.

Homeopathic remedies are based on natural substances, such as herbs, minerals, and bee-stings, and have two important distinguishing features. One is that they use Hahnemann's principle of "like cures like." By taking remedies that would produce similar symptoms in a healthy person, the sick person's immune system is encouraged to fight back. Secondly, and controversially, Homeopathic remedies are so highly diluted ("potentized") that no molecules are left of the original substance. However, its energy is said to remain, and the higher the potency—that is, the more highly diluted the substance is—the more powerful the effect.

Though regarded with scepticism by many orthodox doctors, Homeopathy can be understood in terms of energy. Hahnemann believed that the body contains a "vital force" that regulates good health. Illness is a direct result of the body's attempts to restore order when it has been subjected to disruptive forces such as poor diet and stress. Remedies are prescribed that will work at a vibratory level to encourage healing.

In addition, water has been found to be an excellent hoarder of energy. Recent experiments into Homeopathy suggest that water which is "succussed" (shaken) over and over again at each dilution retains an energy imprint of the original substance.

The correct Homeopathic treatment for a condition should be based on a complete picture of the patient, encompassing physical, mental, and emotional aspects. Different remedies may be given to different people for the same disease. It is therefore always advisable to see

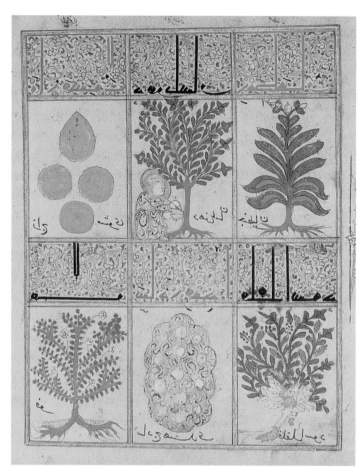

The powerful healing properties of some plants have long been known. This 13th-century Arabic manuscript, the Treatise on the Theriac, *contains paintings of six theriacs or antidotes to poisons.*

a practitioner, or to ask a Homeopathic pharmacist for advice. However, some useful remedies can be kept for First Aid, such as Arnica, Gelsemium, Ignatia, Nux vomica, and Rhus tox. Arnica is used to treat bumps and bruises. Gelsemium can soothe sore throats and pre-exam nerves. Ignatia is valuable for shock and grief. Nux vomica aids hangovers, indigestion, and morning sickness, and Rhus tox can alleviate joint and tendon sprains, rheumatism, and chilblains. All remedies are followed by a number that indicates their potency. Generally, low potencies, such as 6c, are used for mild complaints; higher potencies, such as 30c, are used for more severe complaints.

FLOWER ESSENCES AND REMEDIES

Dr Edward Bach (pronounced "batch"), the pioneer of Flower Remedies, was a Homeopath and physician. He believed that the energy of plants could be used to produce remedies even more gentle than those used by Homeopaths, in order to heal the emotional and spiritual disharmonies underlying physical illness. During the 1930s, he worked intuitively, experimenting on himself, until he produced a range of 38 remedies to deal with various states of mind, including fear, depression, discouragement, lack of confidence, anger, and resentment. His 39th and most famous remedy is a combination of five essences: cherry, plum, clematis, impatiens, rock rose, and star-of-Bethlehem. Known as Rescue Remedy, this combination of essences is said to have a calming and comforting effect.

Bach Flower Remedies are pure energy medicine. As with Homeopathy there is no molecule of the original plant left in the remedy, only its energy. The appropriate flowers for the remedy, organically grown, are picked at their best and their heads floated in a bowl of spring water in sunlight. After several hours the water, energized by the Sun, begins to bubble. The flower heads are removed, and the water is stored in dark bottles, with some brandy as a preservative.

The use of Bach Flower Remedies has spread throughout the world, mainly by word of mouth. In the 1970s a veritable explosion of Flower Remedies and essences appeared on the market, as other flower essence therapists began making their own ranges, usually applying similar methods to Dr Bach's. There are now some 4,000 remedies available, using plants from Africa, the Amazon, Australia, and New Zealand, Alaska, the Himalayas, Hawaii, Yorkshire in England, and Findhorn in Scotland. Flower (and gem and sea) essences

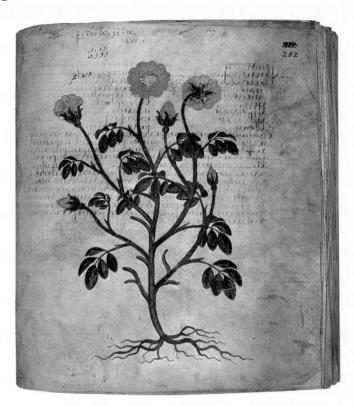

Soothing roses feature in this medical codex, thought to have been produced in Constantinople (Istanbul) in the 6th century.

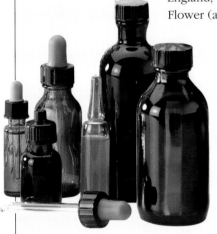

Generally, Flower Remedies are taken in liquid form, by adding a few drops to a glass of water. Store them in dark bottles.

work on the energy system in a gentle, non-invasive way. They aim to treat inner disharmony and negative thoughts and feelings, and can prevent emotional and mental stress from taking root in the body. Most are further diluted, by putting a few drops in a glass of water, and taken by mouth; there are some creams and sprays also available. All the remedies are believed to be safe and can be used on babies, animals, and even plants. It's useful to keep a bottle of Rescue Remedy for emergencies, from accidents to pre-exam stress.

Flower Remedies are safe to prescribe for oneself and are not known to have any contraindications. When selecting the appropriate remedy for your emotional needs, use a guide such as the comprehensive *The Encyclopedia of Flower Remedies* by Clare G. Harvey and Amanda Cochrane. If you pick an inappropriate remedy, it will have no effect. If in doubt, consult a professional flower therapist.

AYURVEDIC MEDICINE

Ayurveda is a Sanskrit word that means the "knowledge or science of life." The Ayurvedic medical system was developed in India 3,000 years ago by a group of *rishis* (spiritually developed humans) who went into deep meditation in order to find the reasons and cures for diseases that affected humans, animals, and plants. Ayurvedic medicine is based on the concept that a universal energy gives life to everything, from the Sun to individual human cells. The body is seen as a microcosm of the universe, governed by complex external and internal energies.

In Ayurveda all matter, whether living or dead, is composed of five elements: earth, water, fire, air, and ether. Each of these elements has its own qualities: the mixture of them in different proportions results in the infinite variety of life on Earth. In our bodies, the five elements are variously combined to form three vital energies, known as the three *doshas*: Vata, Pitta, and Kapha. Each *dosha* is made up of two elements. Vata is ether and air, Pitta is fire and water, Kapha is water and earth. Although the *doshas* permeate the entire body, they are thought of as belonging primarily to certain regions. Vata is the main driving force in the body. It flows through all the bodily passages and plays an active role in the nervous, respiratory, and circulatory systems. It is connected with the colon. Pitta rules fire in the body. Its Western equivalent is digestion and metabolism, and it is linked to the stomach. Kapha is associated with the phlegm, moisture, water, and fat in the body, and is related to the lungs.

During our lives the proportion of *doshas* within us changes. However, maintaining the overall balance of these energies is vital if we are to remain free of disease. The most common causes of imbalance include poor diet and lifestyle, mental and physical injury, environmental problems, hereditary influences, and *karma* (cause and effect from previous lives). Because Ayurvedic doctors study a patient's physical, mental, and emotional state, as well as their environment, Ayurveda can be considered a truly holistic form of medicine.

For thousands of years Ayurveda has been at the heart of medicine in India and Sri Lanka, and today Ayurvedic medicine is a six-year university degree course.

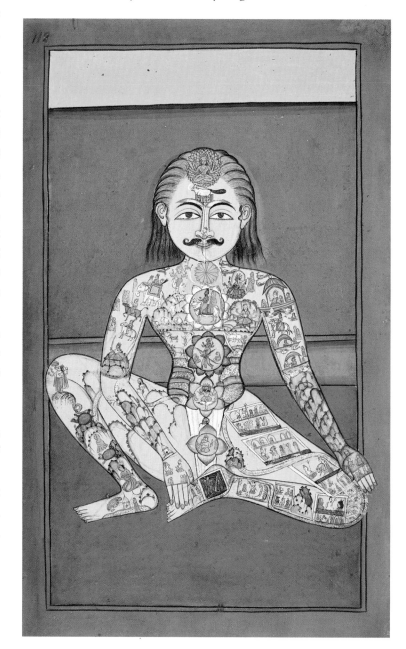

In India, the body is traditionally regarded as a microcosm of the universe, as it is sustained by the same energy that runs through all things. Such a concept is illustrated in this 19th-century Indian miniature of a Yogi as a cosmic figure.

BODY TYPES

Within all individuals the proportion of the three *doshas* (Vata, Pitta, and Kapha) varies, and this determines their physical body type, their mental and emotional profile, and their health. It is very rare for the *doshas* to be equally balanced in a person; usually one or two *doshas* are dominant from conception. During a consult-ation, an Ayurvedic doctor determines the dominant *dosha* in a patient, using criteria such as those in the table below.

Those who have Kapha as their predominant dosha have a slow, steady, and strong pulse that is said to resemble a swan swimming on water.

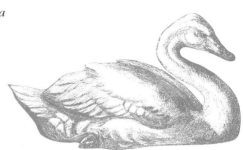

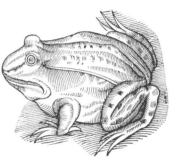

Those people whose body type is predominantly Pitta have an excitable, jumpy pulse, which is likened to the movement of a frog.

CHARACTERISTIC	VATA	PITTA	KAPHA
HEIGHT	Very tall or short	Medium	Often tall
BUILD	Slim	Medium	Heavy
SKIN	Dry and rough	Smooth, freckles	Oily
TEMPERATURE	Cool	Warm	Cold
SWEATS	Little	Moderately	A lot
EYES	Small, gray/black	Small, green/brown	Big, blue
TEETH	Big and crooked	Medium and yellow	Big and white
HAIR	Thin and dark	Thin, red/brown	Thick and dark
PULSE	Fast and irregular	Erratic	Slow and steady
SPEECH	Fast, talkative	Loud, clear	Slow, melodious
APPETITE	Variable	Strong	Moderate
DIGESTION	Good	Strong	Poor
ACTIVITY	High	Moderate	Low
SEX DRIVE	High	Moderate	Low
SLEEP PATTERN	Prone to insomnia	Short and deep	Long and deep
FINANCES	Poor, wastes money	Careful with money	Rich, thrifty
MIND	Creative, artistic	Alert, focused	Steady, reliable
MEMORY	Good short-term, poor long-term	Good	Takes time to retain, but then good

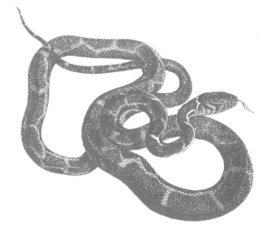

Those with a predominantly Vata constitution possess a thin, quick, and irregular pulse, which is reminiscent of a slithering snake.

AYURVEDIC PRACTICE

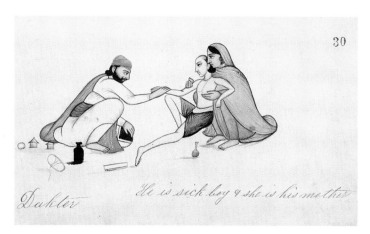

Pulse-taking is one of the primary diagnostic tools of an Ayurvedic practitioner. This watercolor by an East India Company artist dates from around 1860. It depicts a doctor taking the pulse of a sick boy as he lies in the arms of his mother.

Diagnosis in the West usually means the identification of a disease or condition after it has manifested itself. However, an Ayurvedic practitioner will perceive *dosha* imbalances in most people, even those considered to be healthy by a Western doctor. By detecting these imbalances early on, Ayurveda can help to prevent debilitating illnesses from developing.

When you visit an Ayurvedic practitioner, you will be asked for personal details about your family history, lifestyle, dietary habits, and work. Your pulse, tongue, skin, eyes, and nails will be examined in order to find your dominant *dosha* and to look for signs of imbalance. As well as deciding whether their patient has a Vata, Pitta, or Kapha *dosha* by taking their pulse (see page 119), physicians use maps of the face, lips, and tongue to diagnose irregularities in other parts of the body. Cracks in the tongue, for example, can be symptomatic of a problem in the colon, while puffy eyelids could indicate that the kidneys are impaired, and yellow lips may signify jaundice. The nails can also reveal illness, especially

Surgery, such as this eye operation being performed by an oculist, was once performed by Ayurvedic practitioners.

dietary imbalances such as vitamin and mineral deficiencies, while examining the eyes can reveal medical conditions such as diabetes, anaemia, and arthritis as well as heart problems.

Once an Ayurvedic physician has made a diagnosis, he or she will prescribe from a range of possible treatments. These may be taken singly or in combination. Ayurvedic treatments include *marma* therapy, meditation, diet, exercise, oral medications, and *panchakarma*.

According to Ayurveda, there are 107 energy points, known as *marma* points, distributed throughout the

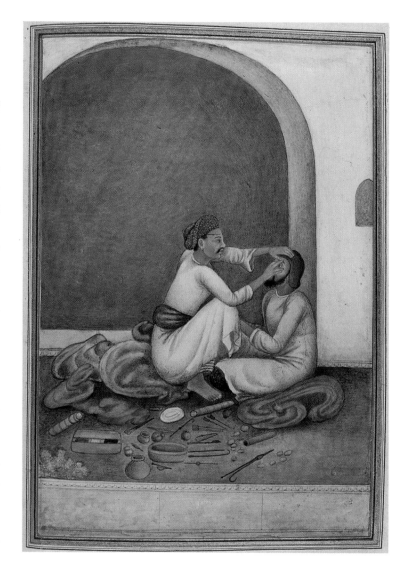

physical body. These points are fed by the energy of the subtle body, which is centered in the chakras (see pages 44–5). There are three main *marma* centers in the body: the head, the heart, and the bladder. Serious injury to any of these centers can cause death.

If the energy at a *marma* point is blocked, there are two main treatments available: *marma* puncture and *marma* massage, which can be compared to the Chinese methods of Acupuncture and Acupressure respectively. *Marma* puncture involves inserting needles, or applying heat with moxa candles to the points. During *marma* massage the points are warmed by the hands. Conditions commonly treated with *marma* therapy include high or low blood pressure, constipation, migraine, sinusitis, impotence, asthma, haemorrhoids, rheumatism, PMS, eczema, irritable bowel disease, and diverticulitis.

Ayurveda is the only medical system in the world to explain in detail the methods of complete cleansing for the prevention and treatment of disease. Although many of the processes may seem alien or unpleasant to those in the West, internal and external cleansing helps the body's energies to flow and the organs to function properly. Five types of cleansing (*panchakarma*) are recommended: inhalations, therapeutic vomiting, herbal enema, oil enema, and laxative administration. Each of these should be undertaken at least once a season to remove excess *doshas* and toxins from the body. Complete or partial *panchakarma* therapy is indicated for most conditions but should be attempted only by an Ayurvedic physician.

Two other cleansing treatments that stimulate the body's energy are *sneha karma* or oil massage, and *sweda karma* or sweat therapy (usually a herbal steam bath). The oil massage brings toxins to the body surface, which are then eliminated from the skin through perspiration during the herbal steam bath. Other techniques include *shirodhara*, in which oil is dripped on the head to aid the brain function, and *rakta mokshana*, or bloodletting, which is recommended by some Ayurvedic experts to purify the blood.

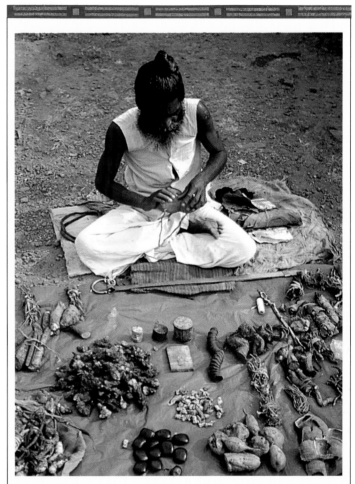

In India, traditional remedies are still sold in their raw, dried form by herbalists on the street.

AYURVEDIC HERBAL MEDICINE

A range of Ayurvedic herbal remedies is available to combat disease and release energy into the body. All the preparations are made from plants, such as coriander, ginger, and jasmine, which have been cultivated for their healing properties for thousands of years. They come in various forms, including essences, powders, poultices, and pills. Traditionally, dried herbs were prescribed by physicians for patients to mix at home. Today, however, medicines are commercially available from qualified practitioners around the world.

EASTERN HERBAL MEDICINES

In the great Oriental medical traditions of China, Japan, and Tibet there has always been a focus on self-care, prevention, and the use of natural therapies to maintain good health. Physicians will normally only recommend surgical and drug treatments as a last resort.

The first steps to health are said to be the development of an awareness of the influence of diet, environment, thoughts, and emotions on the body's energy. It is then necessary to learn how to work positively with each of these factors. If some imbalance still exists then the physician may employ palpation techniques, such as pulse-taking and abdominal diagnosis. The physician will also observe the tongue, skin, and face of the patient, as well as inquiring about any current symptoms. Initial treatment is always based on natural, non-invasive remedies. Each of these ancient medical systems contains a detailed study and practice of herbal medicine.

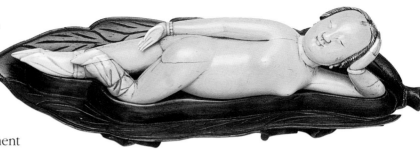

In the 19th century Chinese women were too modest to undress in front of their physician. They therefore used diagnostic figures, such as an ivory doll, to point to the affected area.

Herbs are classified according to their properties and effects on the body's energy. Some are used for cooling the body, as in the case of fever and inflammation, some for warming, and others for cleansing and purging. Different parts of the plant may be used, such as the root, the flower, the leaves, and the bark. Fungi may also be included in herbal prescriptions. The time of picking and

HERBAL DRINKS TO MAKE AT HOME

To warm the body, chop a few slices of fresh ginger and place in a mug together with the juice of half a lemon and a teaspoon of honey. Top up with newly boiled water and sip slowly. You should have a warm sensation throughout your body once you have finished. This is an ideal winter drink that helps prevent and relieve colds, warm the extremities, and ease feelings of nausea.

To cool the body, take four to six medium-sized fresh mint leaves and rinse carefully in cold water. Place in a mug and top up with boiling water. Leave the infusion to stand for five minutes (stir occasionally) then sip. To make a summer drink, mint can be served cold. Mint also clears the head and aids digestion.

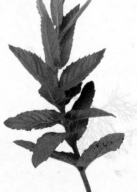

Extracts from ginger, lemon, and mint each have their own energetic affects. If matched to the energy of a patient, these can help to restore health.

the preparation of the herb are both held to be very important. The herbs may be administered in the form of pills, creams, or powders, but very often they are used in their raw form and made into teas or infusions.

Many of the herbs used in Eastern medicines grow in domestic gardens or are available in supermarkets, and are often taken in self-treatment. Cinnamon and ginger, for example, have warming properties and can be added to drinks, cereals, and vegetable dishes to warm the body and promote the flow of energy in the extremities. By contrast, mint is cooling. It stimulates mental activity and aids digestion when made into tea or added to food.

Some of the herbs available for use can be poisonous, so a professional herbalist should always be consulted to approve the use of anything other than culinary herbs. Also, many of the medicines sold by herbalists are derived from shells, minerals, animals, and insects. Patients should always make it clear if they object to taking medicines derived from animal products, especially as these occasionally come from endangered species such as tigers, rhinoceroses, and bears.

Herbal medicine is often combined with other treatments, including massage, Moxibustion (see page 103), and therapeutic exercises from disciplines such as Qigong and T'ai Chi. If all these fail to bring about the desired result, more invasive techniques, such as Acupuncture, blood-letting, and surgery, may be used.

Traditional doctors in China, Japan, and Tibet have always been trained to find and prepare plants and to have a thorough understanding of their medicinal properties. In the West, few doctors nowadays have a wide knowledge of herbal medicines, despite the fact that many drugs, such as aspirin, were once plant-based. This loss of knowledge has contributed to the increasing use in the West of synthetic drugs in place of raw herbs.

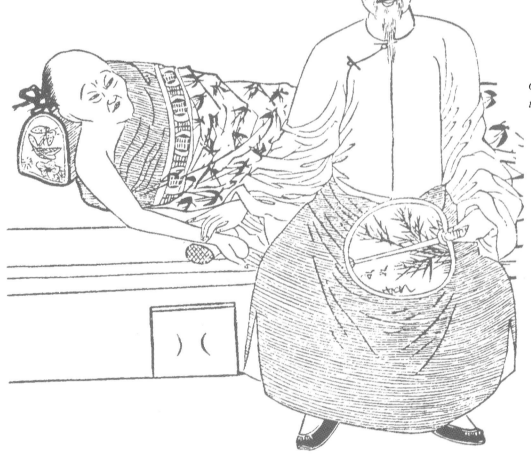

One of the most important diagnostic tools in Chinese Traditional Medicine is pulse-taking. This Chinese wood block, which dates from 1902, depicts a doctor taking his patient's pulse using three fingers.

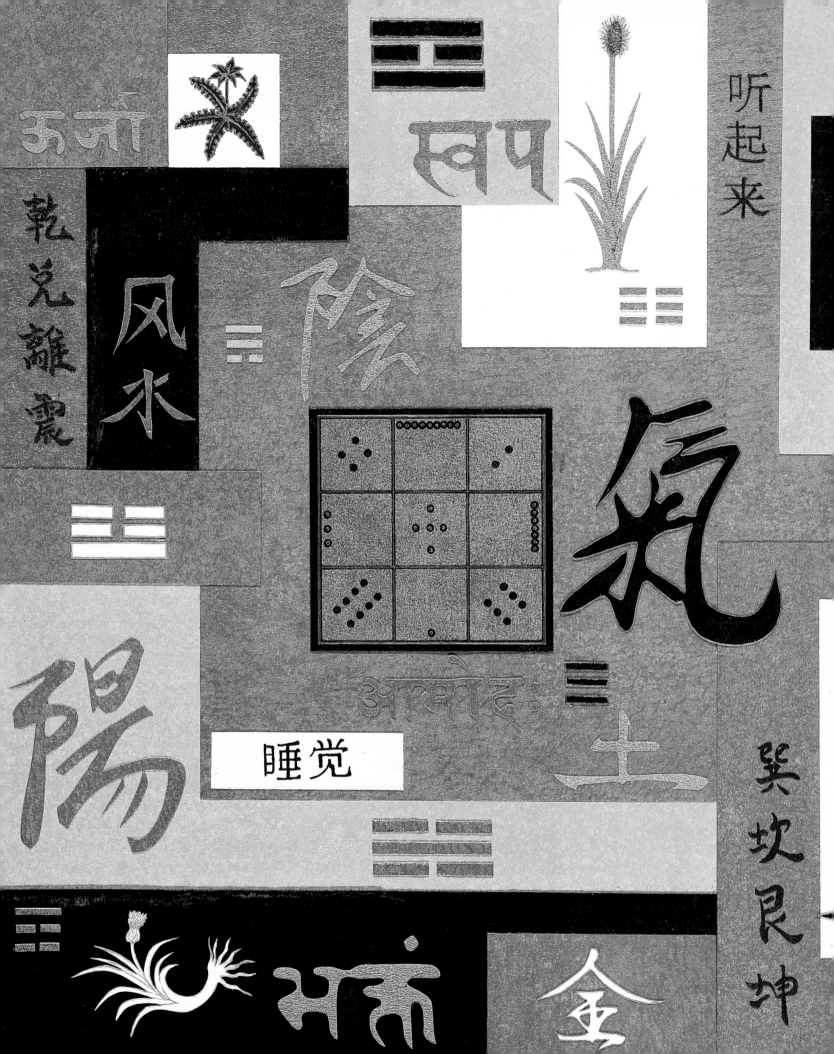

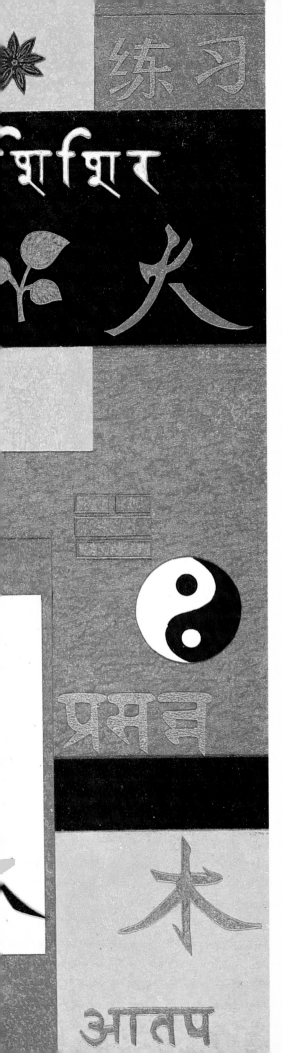

ENERGY, DIET, AND LIVING WELL

Looking after your energy involves every aspect of life: food, drink, work, exercise, and play and, equally importantly, relaxation, rest, and sleep. With today's emphasis on achievement, we often forget the essential need to switch off and replenish our energy. However, Eastern philosophies remind us that the whole is incomplete without both Yin and Yang, darkness and light, activity and rest.

These polarities are reflected in nature's cycles of energy, such as the hours of the day and the four seasons. If we lose touch with these natural rhythms, we do not benefit from energy peaks and cannot defend ourselves from energy troughs.

This chapter shows how to maintain energy and combat stress through diet, relaxation, and sleep, aided by a harmonious environment.

MAXIMIZING YOUR ENERGY

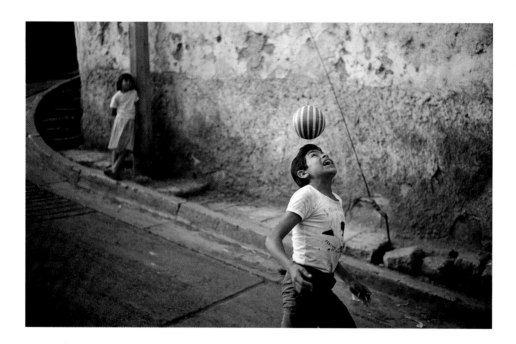

By exercising our imaginations as well as our bodies, and by encouraging laughter, play can make us more healthy.

For our bodies to function properly, we need to eat and breathe well, avoid too much stress, make enough time for relaxation and sleep, and nurture our environment. These factors may rely on the quality of ingredients or technique, but they are also influenced by timing. The digestive system, for example, is at its most efficient early in the morning, becoming less so as the day progresses. Ideally, the main meal should be breakfast or lunch, with a light meal early in the evening.

At certain times our energy needs extra support. In winter, a lack of light can affect the body/mind. Many people suffer from SAD syndrome (Seasonal Affective Disorder) and feel truly depressed and lethargic. Some are helped by sitting for a couple of hours daily in front of a specially designed light-box providing natural daylight. Exercise can also keep the energy flowing, particularly outdoors in daylight.

Extra rest is also vital during illness, pregnancy, and periods of intensive work or emotional stress. "Fighting" illness may be an admirable attitude but should entail cooperating with the body's needs rather than overriding them. Similarly during pregnancy, when a woman is drawing on her own energy to create a new life, she may have to be selfish about her needs. At any stressful period, pay extra attention to nutritional and vitamin requirements, and take plenty of rest. If necessary, seek the help of an alternative therapist, such as a Homeopath.

Just as there is usually a straightforward reason for feelings of tiredness and lethargy, so remedies are often simple and natural. Including 20–40 minutes' walking in your daily schedule (when possible, walking barefoot on sand or grass in the summer) can greatly increase your energy levels. Making time for pleasure can also be very rewarding. Laughter is an instant energizer: it cleanses the solar plexus and sacral chakras. (So does crying, which should not be suppressed if the need arises.)

Energy naturally slows down as we age. We cannot stop the aging process, but we can maintain health and vitality by looking after our energy through good nutrition and exercise. Qigong and Yoga are excellent age combatants; so is walking. Perhaps most important of all is a positive mental outlook: retirement allows time to explore new creative and social activities, and deterioration of the brain cells may slow if you remain active.

DIET AND ENERGY

It has long been known that our diet influences our energy levels. Certain diets can drain and fatigue the body, causing a myriad health problems, while others seem to boost vitality and promote longevity. Sufferers from indigestion or irritable bowel syndrome, for example, often improve when dairy, wheat, and gluten products are excluded from their diet, while those at risk of heart problems are advised to follow a Mediterranean diet with plenty of fresh vegetables, fish, and olive oil in place of saturated fats. Study of the oldest inhabitants on the planet often reveals that they live on a simple, moderate diet of fresh and local food, minimally cooked.

In the West, the emphasis on diet tends to focus on getting a balance between different food groups, such as carbohydrates, proteins, fats, and the food sources of essential vitamins and minerals. Foods are classified according to these groups and recommendations given according to the number of portions required daily. There are also recommended daily allowances for each of the vitamins and minerals essential to health.

A healthy diet is said to be one that contains plenty of fresh fruit and vegetables; complex carbohydrates, such as cereals, wholegrain breads, or pasta; protein in the form of white meat (too much red meat is inadvisable), fish, low-fat dairy products, or pulses; and a small amount of polyunsaturated fats. As more reports about food additives, pesticides, and intensive farming practices emerge, increasing numbers of people are favoring vegetarian and vegan diets and selecting organic foods.

Yet the diet of a large percentage of the population still consists mainly of "junk" food, such as hamburgers, carbonated sugary drinks, processed foods, potato chips, and candy. Eaten in excess, these products can lead to fatigue and ill-health in the long term.

A further problem with Western diets is that, owing to increases in trade and transportation and ways of preserving foods, much of the food consumed is unseasonal and not local. Food is often picked when unripe, refrigerated in transport, and sometimes even irradiated to ensure it has a longer shelf-life. According to Oriental philosophy, these practices rob the food not only of its nutrients but also of its vitality and life energy. This in turn is thought to have an effect on the body's energy because the food is no longer life-enhancing.

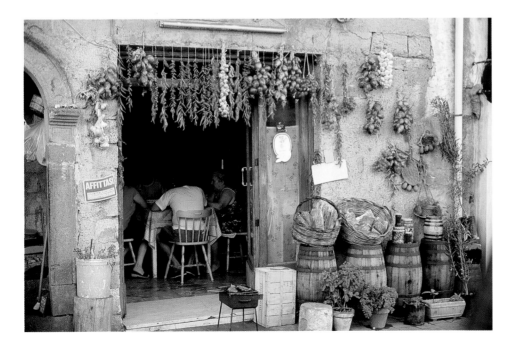

The Mediterranean diet consists largely of fresh fish, vegetables and fruit, garlic, olive oil, and some red wine. It is now being recommended to people with a history of heart disease because it can help to lower the amount of cholesterol in the blood.

THE YIN AND YANG OF FOOD

The Eastern attitude toward food and diet is different from that in the West and is based on an understanding of the properties of foods, and their effects on the body, rather than their actual constituents. All foods can be classified according to the principles of Yin and Yang (see pages 20–21). Basically, foods that demonstrate Yin properties will be cooling, long, thin, watery, soft, and dark in color, while those with Yang properties will be warming, short, broad, dry, hard, and light in color. Typical Yang foods are meat, hard cheese, and salt, while those with Yin characteristics include sugar and alcohol.

In general, aquatic foods, such as fish, shellfish, seaweeds, and algae, tend to be more Yin. Foods from the land are more Yang. Similarly, foods that are grown in the dark or underground, such as root vegetables and mushrooms, are more Yin, while those that grow in the light and above the ground are more Yang. However, these principles are always relative. Fish may be considered Yin because they live in water, but also Yang, compared to seaweed or algae, because they are so active.

Some foods, such as certain grains, are considered "neutral" as they have no overriding warming or cooling property. These neutral foods should form the basis of any diet. The method of cooking is also important and can change the properties of any given food. A piece of fish can be made more Yang by grilling or frying it, while meats, such as chicken, may be made less Yang by steaming them with water rather than frying or grilling.

As they dwell in water, fish are considered Yin, except when compared to less active life forms.

In the Oriental system, a balanced diet should contain plenty of neutral foods and also a balanced intake of Yin and Yang foods. However, it is also vital to adapt the diet according to a person's constitution. Very thin, weak, and cold people, who are excessively Yin, should avoid Yin foods, such as sugar

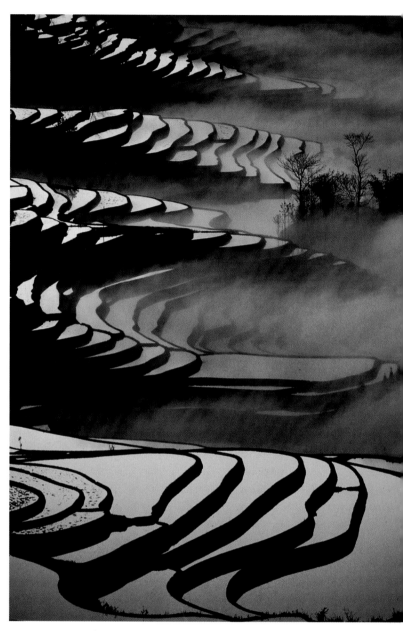

Rice, a neutral food, is the staple of most Eastern diets. It is grown in vast quantities in China, often in terraced paddy fields, such as these in Yunnan.

and alcohol, and ensure a good intake of warming, Yang foods. On the other hand, those who have a tendency to be hot, red-faced, plump, and sweaty should avoid Yang foods, such as meat and cheese, and include more cooling Yin foods in their diet. In this way the body condition can be regulated and diseases can also be controlled, prevented, or even cured.

According to this system of thought, food is not only essential to health and vitality, it is also a crucial factor in the development of the consciousness. Different foods affect the mind and emotions as much as the physical body. Very Yang foods can make a person irritable and aggressive, loud and domineering, restless and hard to please. Very Yin foods can induce lethargy, passivity, and depression. If a person wants to live a long, healthy life, it is essential that he or she eats a modest and balanced diet that avoids extremes. According to the Japanese, the ideal diet to achieve this is a macrobiotic one.

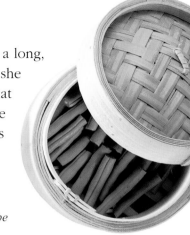

Steaming, a popular way of cooking in the East, increases the amount of moisture in the food, making it more Yin.

MACROBIOTICS

The macrobiotic diet is based on the desire to live in harmony with nature, one's environment, and the universe. It has been used for thousands of years in Japan. Among its principles are: only eating food that is grown locally or in a similar climate; using fresh food; cooking foods lightly and selecting foods in their most natural and whole form.

The diet is described in terms of principal and supplementary foods. At least half of one's daily food should consist of whole grains, such as rice, barley, millet, rye, and buckwheat. These grains, together with pulses such as lentils and kidney beans, are considered the most important foods.

Of the supplementary foods, over half should consist of vegetables grown on the land, while the remaining quarter is principally made up of seeds and seaweeds. The final part of the diet can comprise fruits, seafood, and meat.

Various cooking methods are used, but steaming and grilling are among the most popular. The manner of eating is also important and ranges from presenting the food beautifully to offering it to the gods with gratitude before consumption. Food should be chewed slowly and well and space left in the stomach at the end of each meal.

This 19th-century Japanese print by Kunisada Utagawa demonstrates how eating the wrong foods, or too much of the right foods, can overload the finely tuned digestive system.

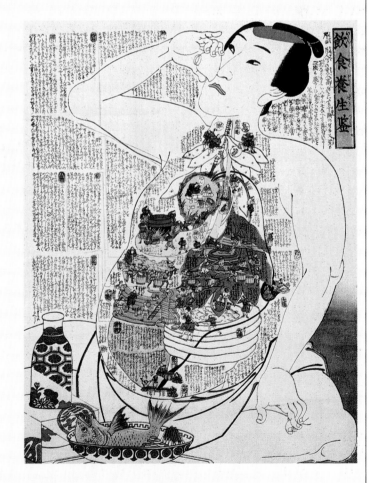

AYURVEDIC THEORIES OF NUTRITION

In Ayurveda, great emphasis is placed on eating the right food in order to prevent disease and enhance vitality. As in the Chinese system (see page 128), food is understood in terms of its inherent nature and its effects on the body, but instead of describing it in terms of two principles—those of Yin (cooling, static properties) and Yang (warming, active properties)—Indian tradition puts each food into one of three broad categories or *gunas*: *rajas, tamas,* and *sattva.* Together, the three *gunas* form the basis of all nature.

Rajasic food is active and energy-enhancing in the physical body, but it is also hot in nature and can stir up emotions. Typical *rajasic* foods are meat. Eating these will tend to make a person aggressive and basically instinctual, so they are best avoided or eaten only in small quantities.

Tamasic food is heavy and phlegmy in nature and tends to make a person feel lethargic and mentally dull. Any food that is old, stale, tinned, processed, or reheated becomes *tamasic* in nature and is also best avoided. Alcohol and cigarettes are also considered to be *tamasic.*

Sattvic food is thought to be ideal because it helps to purify the body and refine consciousness. Typical *sattvic* foods are milk and fruit. Ayurveda recommends that *sattvic* foods should predominate in the diet.

When determining the best diet for people their nature must be taken into account. If they are very *rajasic* (fiery, irritable, and typically suffering from liver and gall bladder problems), then it is essential to remove all *rajasic* foods, such as meat, from their diet and to replace them with *sattvic* foods, including fresh fruit and vegetables. If people are lethargic and *tamasic* in nature, however, they may benefit from eating small amounts of *rajasic* food to heat up the cold, stagnant areas in their bodies and create new vitality.

Sattvic foods are good for those who wish to pursue spiritual practices because of their purifying and consciousness-raising effects, but they should always be considered in the context of their environment. In India—where it is hot and dry much of the time and cows are considered sacred and are well cared for in a natural environment—milk is considered *sattvic* and is a major source of nutrition. However, in Northern European countries such as Britain—where it is often cold and damp and cows may be maltreated, filled with drugs and fearful and suffering when slaughtered—milk can hardly be considered a *sattvic* food. Rather, because of its damp-forming and mucous nature it could even be considered *tamasic,* and may be best avoided.

As well as belonging to one of three *gunas,* foods can be further classified according to their taste (sweet, sour, salty, bitter, astringent, or pungent) and other properties, such as whether they are hot or cold, heavy or light, dry or oily.

The most suitable diet for an individual is best determined by assessing his or her constitutional type according to the three *doshas,* or humors, known as Vata, Pitta, and Kapha. These are manifestations of the five elements (ether, air, fire, water, and earth) in the physical body (see page 118). For example, Vata people—who tend to be thin, weak, and restless—should avoid raw vegetables, dried fruits, very sour foods, and most animal meats, because these foods can stir up this humor and increase their restlessness. Instead they should

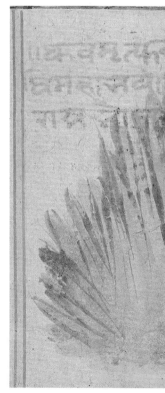

eat plenty of sweet fruits, brown rice, and cooked vegetables. Pitta types—who tend to be strong and eat large quantities—should limit their intake of garlic, onions, peppers, and spices, and eat plenty of green vegetables, salad, apples, and mushrooms. Those with a predominance of Kapha should avoid cold and dairy products and cooling fruits such as bananas, coconuts, or papaya and replace them with dried foods, including dried fruit, white rice, radishes, and pomegranates.

Another important factor in Ayurvedic nutrition is the *agni*, or digestive fire, in the body. If the *agni* is weak, a person's appetite and taste may be poor and he or she may have difficulty in digesting food. Over- or under-eating, or eating poor-quality produce, weakens the *agni* and leads to ill health. Once digested, the food is said to feed the seven *dhatus*, or tissues that make up the body. It is essential to be selective about what you eat; if the *dhatus* are badly nourished, it can lead to both physical and mental disorders.

Ayurveda emphasizes the importance of being calm when eating and recommends that meals are taken in a quiet place, without distractions such as the television. Chew your food thoroughly and leave space in your stomach at the end of a meal. Combining such healthy dietary practices with Yoga exercises, breathing practice, and meditation is said to be the best way to health and spiritual progress.

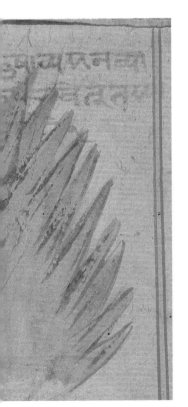

The Sanskrit word agni *means both fire and digestion. It is used to describe the forces present in every cell of the body that break down the substances we consume to release energy.*

WATER

Water plays a vital role in maintaining balance in the body. It should be sipped while eating to moisten the tongue, so that tastes can distinguished more easily, and to aid digestion. Avoid drinking large quantities of water after having eaten, because it will dilute your digestive juices and inhibit the absorption of nutrients. To avoid dehydration, make sure that you vary the amount of water you drink according to the season and temperature.

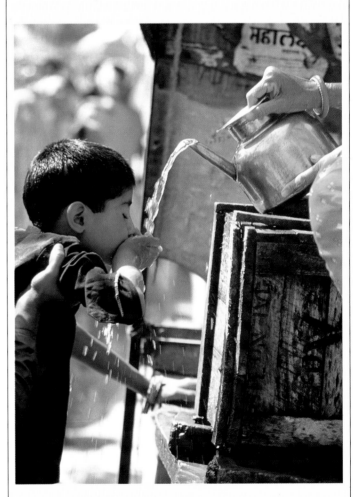

During the summer months, especially in hot climates, make sure that you increase your intake of water.

COPING WITH STRESS

Some stress in our lives can be beneficial: it encourages energy to move around our bodies and enables us to stretch ourselves both physically and mentally. But prolonged, unrelieved stress depletes the immune and nervous systems, making us vulnerable to illness. In general, it is best to prevent stress by following a lifestyle in tune with the natural rhythms of energy. The weekly routine should balance work and chores, exercise, rest, and play.

At work, make sure that you are protected from the electromagnetic pollution emitted from computers and other electrical equipment (see page 150). Watch your posture (see pages 54–5); do not let energy stagnate by sitting too long in one position. During concentrated work or study, take regular short breaks to stretch, breathe, and restore mental energy; try some of the relaxation techniques in this chapter. There is a natural energy dip in the early afternoon when, ideally, a nap would be beneficial. If this is not possible, then take a short walk in the open air. It is also a good idea to avoid important meetings or decisions straight after lunch.

Stress has a direct effect on our breathing patterns. If we are stressed we tend to breathe in quick, shallow breaths. By forcing ourselves to take full, deep, rhythmic breaths when we are under pressure, we can induce a state of calm. Spend more time breathing out than breathing in. The more you breathe out, the more you are able to get rid of the stale air from the respiratory system, and the more you can replace it with fresh air.

Another technique to reduce stress is mentally to replay a pleasant memory or to visualize your favorite view for a few minutes. Using all your senses, recreate every detail of the event or view in your mind's eye.

BREATHING EXERCISE

This breathing exercise increases the circulation of oxygen in the body and helps to relax the muscles. The first part of the exercise expands the chest, allowing more air to enter the lungs. The second part increases the amount of air in the lower part of the chest and uses the palms to focus attention on this area.

After a stressful day at work, use this exercise to clear your mind. Allow the tensions of the day to slip away and focus solely on your breathing. Imagine that with every breath tension is being released and the body and mind are becoming more and more relaxed and peaceful. If performed at the end of the day, this will help to establish a good breathing pattern during sleep too.

Lie down with your arms by your sides. Inhale and stretch both arms above your head. Really feel the stretch as you expand your chest. Exhale, bring your arms back to your sides, and relax. Repeat five times.

Now place your palms against the lower sides of your ribs. Breathe in slowly through your nose, filling the chest from the bottom to the top. As you do this allow the lower chest expansion to push the palms outward. Exhale feeling your palms descend as the lower chest walls subside. Do not hold or strain the breath, but allow it to stay full, deep, rhythmical, and relaxed. Continue this exercise for eight minutes or until you feel completely calm.

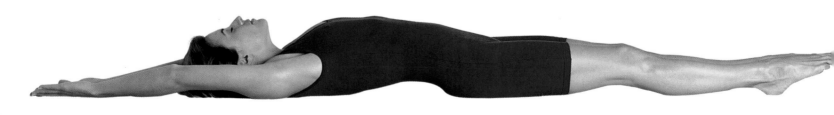

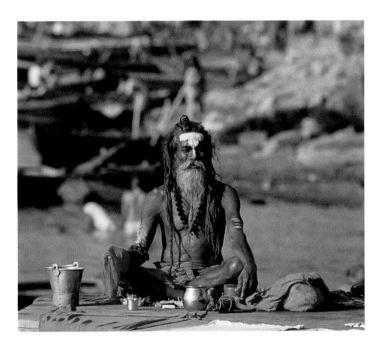

What color was the sky, sea, land? Who was there and what were they wearing? What did they say? What else can you hear? Was there a distinctive smell or taste? Feel the Sun on your face, the texture of the Earth beneath your feet, the wind running through your hair. Enjoy this sensory experience for a few minutes or until you feel relaxed and recharged. Spending time in the serenity of nature is a very important source of relaxation. Images of nature, such as sunrise, sunset, a moonlit night, the sound of the ocean, the countryside, landscapes, a pond or lake are just a few examples.

In Yoga, great emphasis is given to breathing, visualization, and meditation techniques, all of which have been proved to reduce levels of stress. This Yogi is shown meditating on the banks of the River Ganges at Varanasi in India.

CORPSE POSE (SHAVASANA)

Shavasana or the Corpse Pose is the standard Yoga posture for relaxation. It is practiced at the beginning and end of each class, and more briefly between each *asana*. The Corpse Pose is good for releasing physical tension in the body but may also be used to calm the mind. Rather than stretching and then relaxing one part of the body in turn, as suggested here, some schools of Yoga recommend that you extend all your limbs at once in a big stretch.

Breathe from your abdomen (if necessary, place your hands on your abdomen to check that you are breathing correctly). This exercise is usually concluded with the visualization of a happy experience in life—happy memories can be very nourishing.

Lie flat on your back, with your hands about 6 inches (12 cm) from your sides, palms facing upward, and your feet about 12 inches (25 cm) apart. Make sure that your body is perfectly balanced and aligned. Close your eyes and breathe deeply.

Work into the pose by stretching your legs or rotating your ankles and then relaxing them so that your feet are turned slightly outward. Repeat this process of stretching and relaxing arms, head, and any other part of your body that feels tense.

Imagine that your body is limp and heavy and that it is sinking into the ground. Allow yourself to be pulled into the Earth several times. Feel like a child lying securely in the lap of Mother Earth.

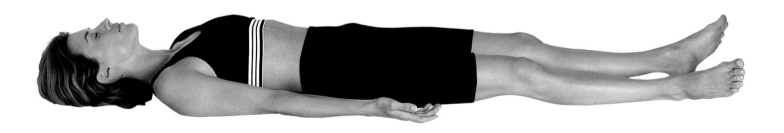

YOGIC MEDITATION

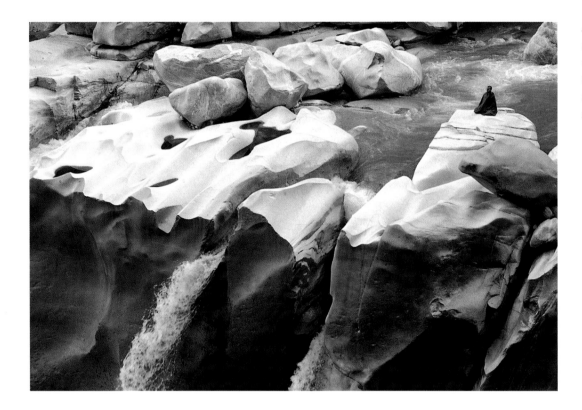

Many people find it easier to meditate outdoors. The River Ganges is particularly sacred to Hindus, and Gangotri on the upper Ganges is a favored site for meditation.

Meditation is a natural state that is obtained by remaining physically still and focusing the mind on one point. This enables the mind to stop chattering, so that intuition may take over and self-revelation gradually develop.

Prepare yourself and your environment well before you begin to practice meditation. Reserve an exclusive place in your home that is quiet, warm, and comfortable. You may wish to build an altar. Cover a table with a piece of white cloth (white symbolizes purity and is a synthesis of all the colors of the spectrum) and decorate it with candles, a picture of a deity, a spiritual symbol, or a vase of flowers. The atmosphere can also be enhanced by burning incense, playing soft, soothing music (such as chants), and dimming the lights.

It is important to meditate at the same time every day. Dawn and dusk are the most spiritually-energetic times, but if these are not practical then choose a convenient time. Begin by meditating for about 20 minutes a day and increase this gradually until you are up to one hour.

Make sure that you are sitting comfortably, adopting a position such as the lotus (see pages 136–7) or simply sitting cross legged or on your heels. Now begin to regulate your breathing. Inhale and exhale deeply for a few minutes and then consciously begin to slow it down. Remember to breathe solely through your nose, to increase the amount of oxygen in your blood and helps to regulate the flow of Prana through your body (see pages 42–3).

Now, without fidgeting, concentrate on a physical object—such as a lighted candle, sacred symbol, or flower—to the exclusion of everything else. Initially, you should allow yourself a small amount of variety in the object you choose. For example, rather than meditating on a flower, choose a whole plant. When you feel tired of gazing at the flower, you can rest your eyes by looking at the leaves and stem before returning to the flower.

Meditating on a sacred symbol such as OM (see page 41), a cross, a lotus, or a yantra (a geometrical diagram)

TRATAK

Practicing tratak involves gazing at an object or point without blinking. When performing tratak you should keep your body absolutely still, so that only your optical nerves are active.

Tratak is usually performed looking at the flame of a candle, but other objects can be used, such as the symbol OM (see page 41), the image of a deity, a flower, the tip of the nose, and the space between the eyebrows.

Place the object of concentration at eye level an arm's length away from your body. Look at it steadily, without straining your eyes. When your eyes feel tired and start watering, gently close them. Now imagine that the object of concentration has reappeared in your third eye or heart region.

When the mental image gradually vanishes, open your eyes and start gazing again. The gazing time can gradually be increased with practice.

Tratak is also used as one of the six cleansing techniques, or Shat Kriyas, used in the Hatha Yoga tradition. The others are nasal cleansing, colon cleansing, stomach cleansing, abdominal churning, and respiratory system cleansing. Tratak strengthens the optical nerves and improves the eyesight.

Hatha Yoga has placed great emphasis on tratak. It gradually purifies and stills the mind, and is a very good exercise for developing the concentration. Initially it influences the optical nerves through the concentration of vision. Gradually it starts gaining control of the external senses,

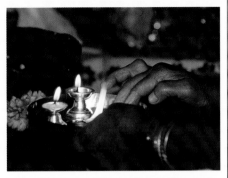

Although any object can be the focus of attention, tratak is most commonly practiced gazing at a candle flame.

leading to trance and higher states of awareness. With practice, the distracting influence of the senses begins to diminish and revelation takes place.

helps you to become aware of the symbol's profound spiritual meaning. All of the above are symbols of the Absolute, the origin of all things. Meditating on such a symbol gives a sense of unification with others in the universe and with the Absolute. It underlines the omnipresent reality.

Once you are able to concentrate on an external object, bring your mind to rest on an internal focal point, such as your Ajna chakra (brow center) or Anahata chakra (heart center). Make sure that you always return to the same focal point when you meditate.

Alternatively, close your eyes and visualize a sacred symbol. You may find that your concentration is aided by repeating a mantra (see page 41) silently or out loud. Even if you do not manage to enter a meditative state at first, you are still conditioning your mind positively. Keep practicing and you will find that your powers of concentration improve and eventually you will be able to enter superconsciousness.

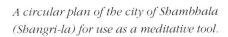

A circular plan of the city of Shambhala (Shangri-la) for use as a meditative tool.

TIBETAN RELAXATION SKILLS

In traditional Tibetan medicine the body's energy is said to be determined by the balance of three "humors": wind, bile, and phlegm. These humors exist in all things and regulate the organ function of the human body. Each humor can be influenced by factors such as diet, environment, and even mental attitude, and disease is said to occur when there is an imbalance in the three humors.

There are three main types of stress recognized by Tibetan medicine, all of which relate to the three humors. Wind is related to respiration and movement, and wind stress is characterized by mental agitation, tension, tiredness, ringing in the ears, and constipation. Bile is linked to digestion, the complexion, and the temperament, so bile stress is characterized by indigestion, irritability and impatience, headaches and migraine. Because phlegm is related to sleep, mobility, and flexibility, phlegm stress is linked to insomnia, dullness, depression, lethargy, fatigue, and cold extremities.

In order to balance the humors one's diet and exercise should be moderate, the climate mild, the level of work reasonable, and the mental attitude positive. One's actions are also held to be important, and a life of non-violence, charity, and compassion is held to be the basis for good health and longevity.

Mental and emotional attitudes play a key role in maintaining balance. Buddhist medicine classifies three mental poisons that influence the three humors in the body and therefore underlie all disorders. Desire, including covertness, envy, and attachment, creates wind disorders. Hatred, incorporating anger and jealousy, promotes bile imbalance. Ignorance, in the form of mental laziness, confusion, and misunderstanding, increases phlegm. A conscious effort should be made to keep the three poisons out of the body.

The key to body balance is through relaxation. This allows the individual to heal and rejuvenate, and also to link with the unseen, yet limitless, vitality of the universe. As the body becomes relaxed the humors are more balanced and the mind becomes calm and alert.

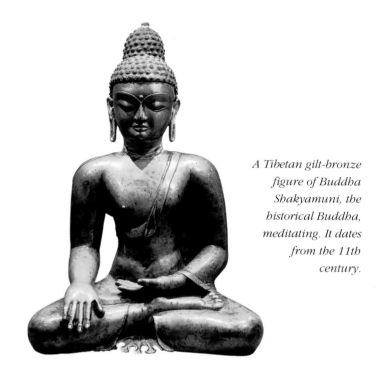

A Tibetan gilt-bronze figure of Buddha Shakyamuni, the historical Buddha, meditating. It dates from the 11th century.

BUDDHIST MEDITATIONAL POSE

The most effective way to relax is through regular practice of a comfortable, meditational sitting posture. In the traditional Buddhist meditation pose, both mind and body become relaxed and the body's energy flow becomes smooth and regular. The pose has seven special features.

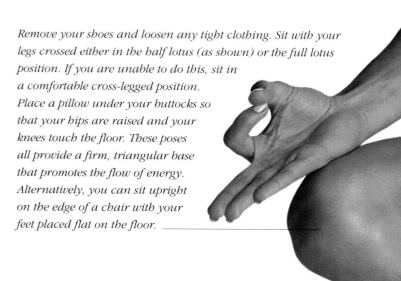

Remove your shoes and loosen any tight clothing. Sit with your legs crossed either in the half lotus (as shown) or the full lotus position. If you are unable to do this, sit in a comfortable cross-legged position. Place a pillow under your buttocks so that your hips are raised and your knees touch the floor. These poses all provide a firm, triangular base that promotes the flow of energy. Alternatively, you can sit upright on the edge of a chair with your feet placed flat on the floor.

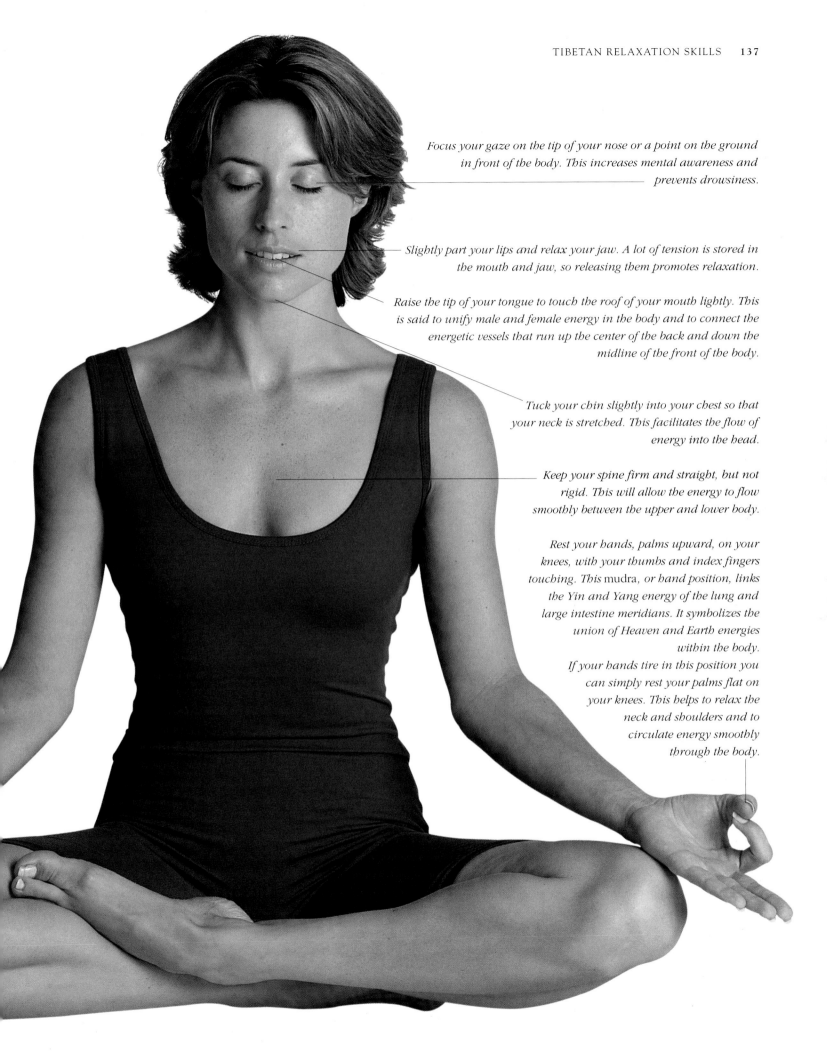

Focus your gaze on the tip of your nose or a point on the ground in front of the body. This increases mental awareness and prevents drowsiness.

Slightly part your lips and relax your jaw. A lot of tension is stored in the mouth and jaw, so releasing them promotes relaxation.

Raise the tip of your tongue to touch the roof of your mouth lightly. This is said to unify male and female energy in the body and to connect the energetic vessels that run up the center of the back and down the midline of the front of the body.

Tuck your chin slightly into your chest so that your neck is stretched. This facilitates the flow of energy into the head.

Keep your spine firm and straight, but not rigid. This will allow the energy to flow smoothly between the upper and lower body.

Rest your hands, palms upward, on your knees, with your thumbs and index fingers touching. This mudra, or hand position, links the Yin and Yang energy of the lung and large intestine meridians. It symbolizes the union of Heaven and Earth energies within the body.
If your hands tire in this position you can simply rest your palms flat on your knees. This helps to relax the neck and shoulders and to circulate energy smoothly through the body.

QIGONG RELAXATION TECHNIQUES

To relax and open up the body is one of the key aims of Qigong practice. As you progress and go deeper into a Qi state, you will notice that your natural breathing pattern changes. It may become deeper, slower, and more smooth. At a certain stage you should expect your breathing to feel as if it is coming from the abdomen rather than from the chest. This helps to relieve tension in the chest and shoulders.

RELAXING THE NECK AND SHOULDERS

The neck and shoulders are two of the most abused areas of our body. Their muscles become hunched when we are stressed, and strained every time we carry a heavy bag or sit awkwardly. This exercise is designed to release tension in your neck and shoulders and to take the energies down to your feet. Remember to be conscious of the inside of your body, rather than looking outward.

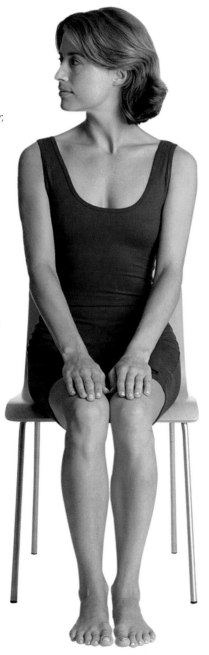

1 *Sit on the edge of a chair, back straight, with your feet firmly on the ground parallel, and together. Drop your shoulders and rest your hands gently on your knees.*

  Smoothly turn your head to the right, then back to the center, then left and back to the center. Repeat ten times.

  Still keeping your feet flat on the ground and together, swivel your heels from side to side as far as you can. Repeat ten times.

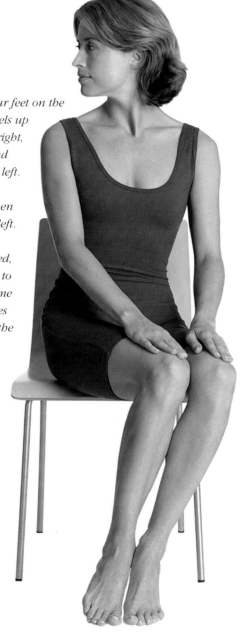

2 *With the balls of your feet on the ground, lift your heels up and move them to the right, down to the ground and then swivel them to the left. Continue this rotating movement ten times, then repeat ten times to the left.*

  Then, with your feet together and heels raised, slowly move your head to the right at the same time as you swivel your knees to the left. Now stretch the other side (head to the left, knees to the right). Repeat ten times.

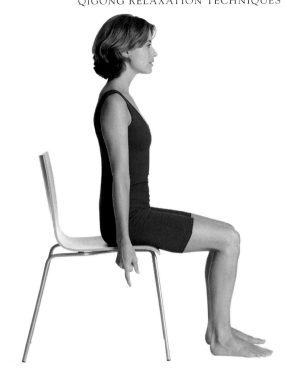

SITTING DOWN BREATHING EXERCISE

This exercise is designed to quieten the brain and loosen the stress in the shoulders. It is excellent if you come home tired and need to be revitalized, before continuing with more exercises.

Sit on the edge of a chair. Put both feet on the ground, parallel and a hips' width apart. Drop your shoulders and let your arms hang by your sides. Bend the last three fingers on each hand, allowing the thumbs and index fingers to form a "V" that points upward. Breathe in through your nose, but imagine you are breathing in through the top of your head. Exhale gently through your mouth, but imagine you are breathing out through your fingers and thumbs. Repeat for 15 minutes, then shake your hands and gently shake your head until you feel completely clear.

LYING DOWN BREATHING EXERCISE

Deep breathing techniques are used by many disciplines actively to reduce stress and to calm the mind. This exercise not only relaxes the body, but it also encourages its vital energy to flow freely from the head to the feet.

Lie on your back with your hands loosely placed one on top of the other over your lower abdomen. Position your feet so that your toes are together and your heels are apart. Allow the focus of attention to be on your heels—imagine when breathing in and out that the air reaches your heels. Stay in this position for five minutes or until you feel as if your whole body is breathing from the heels.

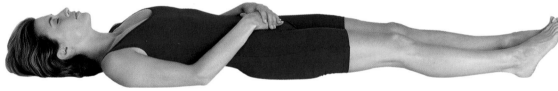

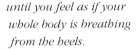

STRENGTHENING THE KIDNEYS

This exercise strengthens the kidneys, which are two of the most important organs in Chinese medicine, because they store Congenital or Pre-Heaven Qi (see page 16). Each kidney could fit into the palm of the hand and is located on either side of the spine, just above the waist, behind the lower ribs.

Lie on your back on the floor. Bend your right leg up and outward so that your foot rests by your left knee. Place your left hand under the back with the palm facing the left kidney. Place your right hand over your navel. Imagine that your left hand is warming the left kidney and that the energy of your right hand is piercing your navel and penetrating through your body to your left kidney.

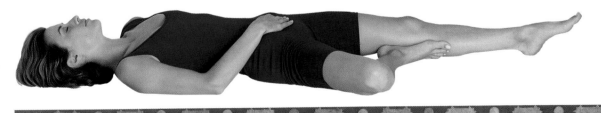

SELF-MASSAGE

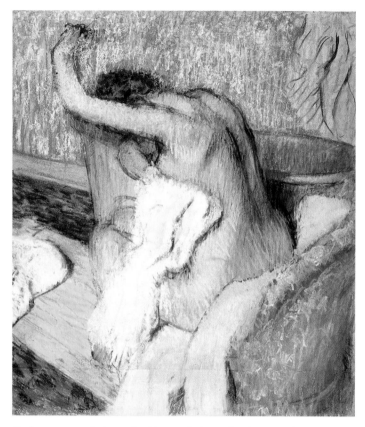

Today, we rarely have the time or privacy to give ourselves a loving, unhurried massage, such as that evoked by After the Bath, Woman Drying Herself, *painted c.1889 by Edgar Degas.*

One of the best ways of calming your nerves, releasing stress, and encouraging a general feeling of well-being is through self-massage. By lavishing attention, care, and time on yourself, you are investing in your health and happiness. In an age when an increasing number of women, men, and even children profess to dislike their own bodies, self-massage can help to create an acceptance and love of the way we look and feel.

There are many detailed books on self-massage, showing different techniques and practices. However, the most valuable technique in self-massage is impossible to learn from others. It is only by tuning in to our own sensations—giving to and receiving from ourselves—that we increase our own well-being and achieve relaxation.

After all, nobody knows as well as we do ourselves what pressure feels good, or what spot relieves an ache.

To achieve a truly healing self-massage, you need to put into practice all the awareness methods you have learned to use on another person (see pages 77–97). Be aware of your breathing, of your contact with the ground, of your energy field around you. Tune in to the sensations of your whole body, not just the part you are working on. And most importantly, relax!

If you have the time, it is a good idea to prepare for a self-massage by taking an aromatic bath. This is particularly relaxing if you bathe by candlelight, listening to some music that inspires you. Lie in the bath with your eyes closed, inhale the essences, and enjoy the warmth of the surrounding water. Have a warm, fluffy towel ready to dry yourself with when you get out.

Mix yourself some scented oil, collect some towels and cushions, and find somewhere warm, comfortable, and quiet. Dim the lights (or use candles), listen to music, and either burn incense or heat essential oils to scent the air. Take a few deep breaths to relax.

Sit on a towel on the floor or a chair, using cushions for support if necessary. It is essential that you are comfortable. You should be able to reach almost every part of your face and body, with the possible exception of your middle back, but do not strain or force yourself. Listen to the richness of your sensations, the unique sensitivity of every part of you and what it tells you, where it leads.

Pour a small amount of oil onto your hands and then begin the massage by exploring your face with sensitivity. Keep tuning in to your whole body and relaxing your breathing. If a stroke feels good, repeat it several times to get a sense of rhythm. Listen to your sensations. Massage your whole body right down to your toes. Pay attention to your body's needs: if your hands get tired, rest, or try using your elbows instead. Elbows can feel wonderful sliding slowly along oiled skin.

If we can occasionally make the time for ourselves, a massage can be memorable and rewarding.

MASSAGING YOUR HANDS

For an instant stress-reliever try massaging your hands. Once again, what is important is not so much the massage but the quality of awareness that you bring to it, so relax your breathing, be aware of your feet on the floor, and tune in to the sensations of your whole body. Let both hands rest on your lap for support.

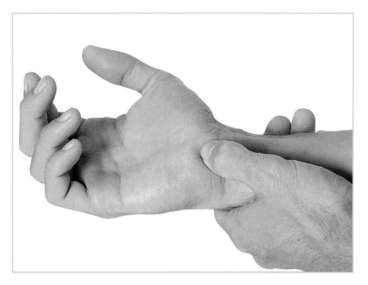

2 *Turn your hand palm upward and hold your wrist between the thumb and fingers of the other hand. Massage the wrist and the base of the palm with your thumb tip, supporting the wrist with your fingers. Now massage the entire palm in deep circular movements, supporting the back of your hand with your fingers.*

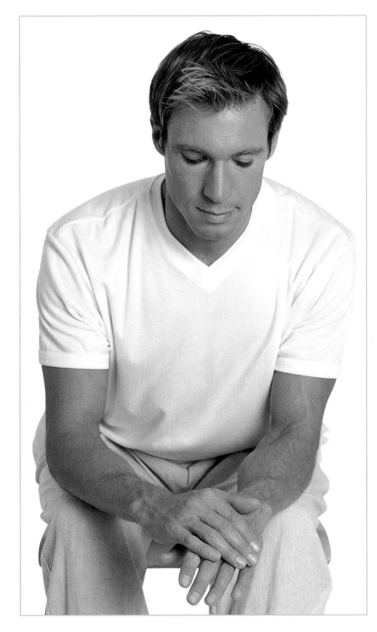

1 *Leaning your elbows on your thighs, stroke one of your hands, front and back, including the wrist. Relax the giving hand and mold it to the contours of the receiving hand.*

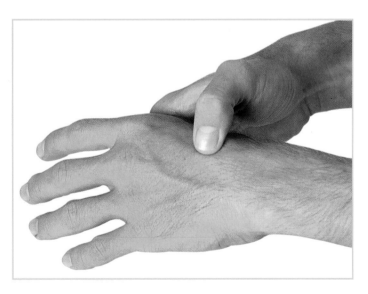

3 *Now turn your hand over and massage the back of the wrist and hand. Using small circular movements work between the bones of the back of the hand, from wrist to knuckles. Support the palm with your fingers and keep your shoulders and arms relaxed.*
  Now massage each finger and both thumbs in turn, following the Shiatsu finger massage on page 37.

USING KINESIOLOGY TO REDUCE STRESS

In the modern, fast-moving world most of us suffer from stress and do not have enough time to relax. Kinesiology offers a very fast, effective, and powerful technique for releasing stress and bringing about a feeling of deep relaxation. Its system of muscle testing demonstrates the effect of emotional stress on the body and its energies. The meridians most affected by emotional stress are connected with the brain and the stomach—we all know the feeling of butterflies in the stomach when we are very tense. The Kinesiology technique to reduce stress in the body involves activating reflexes that balance these two meridians. New imaging technology used in medical research to record brain activity has revealed specific areas of the brain that are connected with emotional circuits and can be treated to reduce stress. Interestingly, these are in the same location as the reflexes used in Kinesiology to release emotional stress.

Stress has an impact upon the whole body, its emotions and its energy, and in seeking to reduce tension in one area we must address the others.

REDUCING PHYSICAL STRESS: STIMULATING THE IMMUNE SYSTEM

A variety of conditions, from asthma to allergies, are increasingly being blamed on a stressed immune system. A key part of our body's defence mechanism is the thymus gland, which produces T-lymphocytes that stimulate the body to fight infections. It is located in the middle of the upper chest behind the breastbone. The thymus gland is also part of the endocrine system and is connected to the heart energy. It is affected by emotions, so that when a person feels stressed it shrinks and when he or she feels loved it enlarges. Its size can change dramatically in as little as 24 hours, which could explain why people often get ill after a period of extreme stress and why other people look healthy and radiant when they are in a loving relationship.

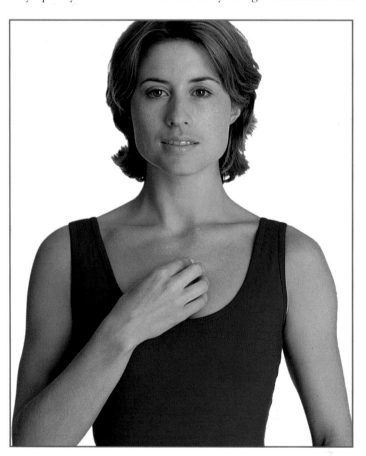

Kinesiology testing can evaluate the energy of the thymus gland and uses the following, simple exercise to stimulate it. This also has the effect of balancing the energies in the body at least for a short period of time. So anything that we can do to improve the function of this gland is helpful to the whole body.

Place all your fingers and both thumbs together on your breast bone in the upper part of your chest. Tap this area to a waltz rhythm for about 20 seconds. You may repeat this as often as you wish.

EXERCISE TO RELIEVE EMOTIONAL STRESS

When a person becomes stressed, the blood supply is drawn away from the peripheral areas of the skull and redirected to the large muscles of the body. This is a primitive response, enabling us to respond immediately to danger. It would have been used by our earliest ancestors when fleeing from predators or fighting a bear at the cave entrance. However, the stresses we encounter today rarely require such direct physical response; we are more often required to behave in a controlled way that conceals how we really feel. We still experience, however, the chemical changes that take place in our body during moments of stress.

The reflexes Kinesiologists use to relieve stress are located on the brow midway above the eyebrows where we can sometimes feel slight bumps. These two reflexes seem to connect energetically with the right and left hemispheres (frontal lobes) of the brain. When they are activated by very light touch, they attract the blood supply back to these areas. The frontal lobes are where our higher thinking centers are located and are the parts of the brain that are active during meditation. If we activate these centers when we are feeling emotionally stressed, we activate a part of the brain that can process the emotionally charged material in a different way. The result is that, although the original stress has not changed, the way in which we perceive and experience it alters—which is why people often report that they no longer feel upset.

Close your eyes and place your fingertips lightly on two points that are located midway between your eyebrows and the natural hair line above your eyes. Concentrate on the situation or issue that is causing you to feel stressed. Experience it as fully as possible, being aware of what you see, hear, feel, taste, and smell. Repeat the process a few times until you find it difficult to continue to think about it. Open your eyes and be aware of how you feel when you think about it now.

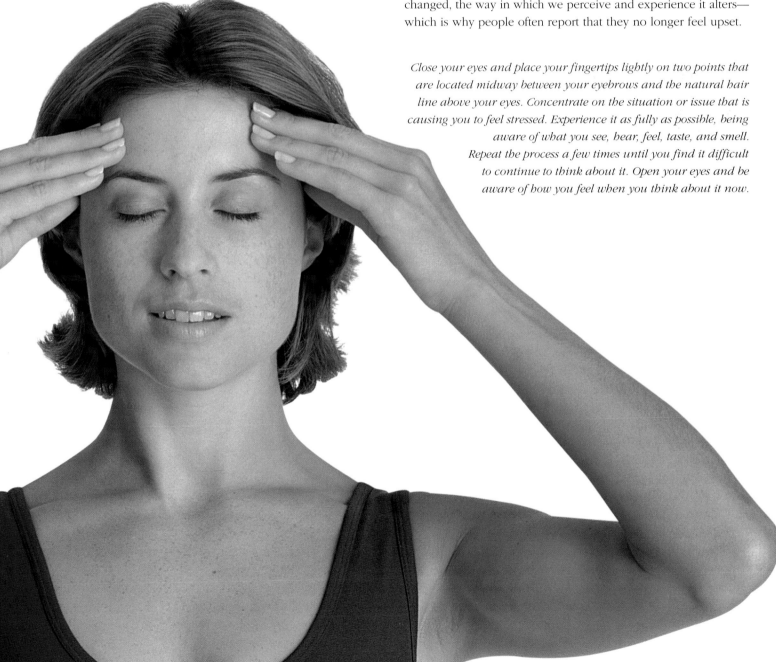

SLEEP

Sleep is essential to maintaining energy. It rests not only the body, but also the mind. Dreaming helps to sort out the day's events, while deep or core sleep gives the brain complete rest. If we eat well, exercise regularly, and enjoy life, good sleep should come about naturally. Individual sleep requirements vary between five and ten hours; do not constantly try to take less than you need. (Dozing off easily during the day may be a sign of insufficient sleep.) However, taking time to relax and meditate daily often diminishes sleep needs. Make sure that you wind down toward bedtime—avoid vigorous exercise, arguments, stimulants, or heavy meals late in the evening.

ACUPRESSURE

Acupressure (see pages 104–5) can be a very useful method of relieving insomnia and promoting a good night's sleep. One of the most powerful points to use is Heart 7, which is located on the wrist. This point calms the mind and aids relaxation. Acupressure to the point Conception Vessel 17, located in the middle of the breastbone in line with the nipples, can also be helpful. This point opens the chest and improves breathing.

If you suffer from insomnia, apply pressure to one of the suggested acupoints one hour before you go to bed and then again just before you go to sleep. It works particularly well when used in combination with a breathing exercise, such as that shown on page 132. Train yourself to follow a regular sleep pattern by repeating the Acupressure technique daily for four to six weeks. Thereafter, use it whenever you are unable to sleep.

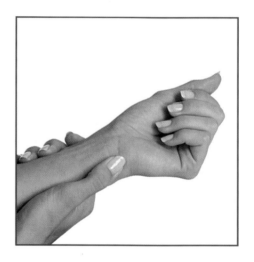

Heart 7 is located on the inside wrist, level with the little finger, just behind the wrist crease. Support your wrist with your fingers and apply pressure with your thumb angled toward the little finger. Press and release for 60 seconds. Repeat on the other wrist.

SLEEP POSITION

Your position can affect the quality of your sleep. Make sure that the energy in your bedroom is harmonious (see page 149) and that there are no electrical appliances near you. To conserve energy, try adopting this position recommended by Zhixing Wang.

Lie on your right side for preference, with your right leg straight and your left bent. Place your left foot behind your right knee, your left hand over your left hip joint, and your right hand beside your head. Your left knee should rest on the bed and your left shoulder should open out slightly toward the back.

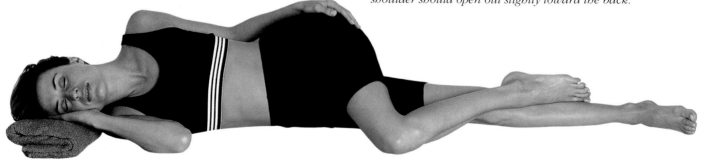

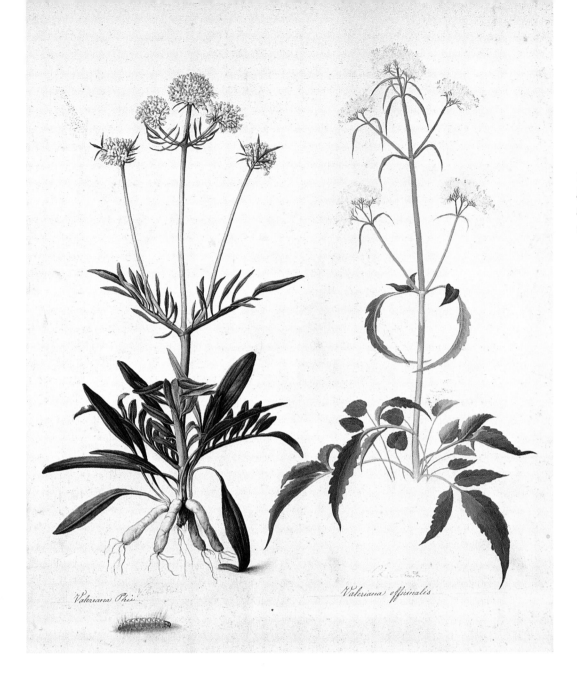

Valeriana Ohie

Valeriana officinalis

The herb valerian is well known for its ability to calm the nerves and combat restlessness and insomnia.

HERBAL REMEDIES

The plant valerian has been used for centuries to aid relaxation and sleep. Infuse about 1 oz (28 g) of dried leaves in 1 pint (600 ml) of freshly boiled water for a few minutes, strain, and drink in the evening before sleeping. Other good herbs for relaxing teas include camomile and passion flower. Many of these herbs are also available in pill or liquid-tincture form in over-the-counter remedies. One very effective herbal ingredient taken mostly in supplement form is kava kava, which is the root of a plant from Polynesia. To be effective, however, it needs to be taken regularly at bedtime for four to six weeks as its effect builds up over time.

Herbs can also be used to make wonderfully relaxing baths that prepare you for sleep. To make them yourself simply infuse the leaves of any of the above-mentioned herbs in a jug or teapot of boiling water. Leave to stand for ten minutes, strain, and add to the bath. Alternatively, tie the dried leaves and flowers in a muslin bag and hang it from the taps in the bath. Take care not to have the bath water too hot and do not soak longer than 20 minutes. Go straight to bed after the bath is finished.

The traditional hop pillow is also an effective remedy for sleep problems—the hops have a slightly soporific effect. However, some people may be allergic to hops, so care must be exercised. Adding a drop of an aromatherapy oil to your own pillow, or using an aromatherapy diffuser in your bedroom, can have a sedative and relaxing effect. The best oils to use are lavender and vetiver, although camomile and rose can also help. The oils can also be massaged into the body (add five drops to about 4 teaspoons (20 ml) of a carrier oil such as sweet almond) or added to bath water (five to ten drops to warm bath water, circulate well).

THE PRINCIPLES OF FENG SHUI

 Feng Shui, pronounced "fung shway," is the art of arranging one's life in accordance with the forces of the universe. It has been practiced by the Chinese for several thousands of years to achieve optimum health and prosperity. Historically, people would search the forests, hills, and plains in order to find the most propitious place on which to build. They would study the Sun, the shadows, and the directions, and once they had chosen a site they would ceremonially choose the date for the work to start.

The majority of early Feng Shui literature focused on finding the appropriate site for burial. Although this aspect of Feng Shui is less relevant today, the principles stated in these classics still apply. In one book, Master Guo Pu asserts: "To bury is to take advantage of the Sheng Qi (Alive Energy). The Qi moves when it meets Feng (Wind) and gathers when it meets Shui (Water). The ancient people would try to make it stay, but not stagnate, to flow but not dissipate. That is why it is called Feng Shui." This statement has been taken by Feng Shui practitioners and scholars to be the authentic definition and the origin of the Feng Shui concept.

As we can see from this definition of Feng Shui, Feng means wind and Shui means water. The circulation of wind (or air) and water symbolizes the natural elements. The energy, or Qi field, is the focus of Feng Shui practice.

In ancient times Feng Shui was also referred to as "The Black Bird Craft." Black Bird was the name given to the officer at the emperor's court who was in charge of geology and astrology. One explanation for this title is that early peoples noticed that the flight path of the black birds along the river was the line of least resistance, where it was most favorable to build houses.

Feng Shui is the art of balancing the environmental elements to create a harmonious Qi field. Wind is the moving, strong, firm Yang aspect. It is represented by mountains in the landscape, which should be behind or supporting a building. Water is the more static, soft, far-reaching Yin aspect. It is represented in the landscape

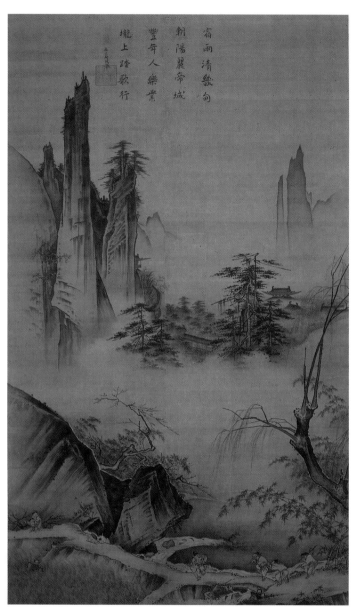

Landscapes, such as this Chinese painting of Willows and Distant Mountains *by Ma Yuan, can be analyzed by Feng Shui masters in terms of their Yin and Yang energies.*

by rivers and lakes, which should be in front of—and not too close to—a building. Balancing the Yin and the Yang aspects utilizes or creates a harmonious Qi field in which to live or work. The Qi is therefore the deciding factor as to whether the Feng Shui of a place is good or not.

TWO SCHOOLS OF PRACTICE

There are two main schools of Feng Shui. The Form School concentrates on the physical formation and structure of a building. The second school uses a sophisticated geomantic compass known as a Luo Pan. This normally has two plates, one representing Heaven and the other representing the Earth. In the middle is a needle that points to magnetic North. Once aligned, readings can be taking from several concentric rings on the compass.

If the Luo Pan is the hardware used by practitioners of the second school, their software is contained in the ancient Chinese book of divination, the *Yi Jing* (*I Ching* or *Book of Changes*, which elaborates Yin-Yang theory) and five-element theory. Both of these systems were developed about 2,000–3,000 years ago and have continued to guide traditional Chinese thought to the present day.

Recently, it has become more difficult to differentiate between the two schools of Feng Shui, because many practitioners have tried to combine the knowledge and methods of both traditions.

A Luo Pan is used to locate the magnetic North Pole. Once the compass is aligned, a master can read off information on the site's energy as well as planetary and calendrical data.

ANIMAL SPIRITS

To the ancient Chinese, the landscape was believed to be alive with spirits, in particular those of known and imaginary animals. A mountain range, with its strong energy, was therefore known as the Long Mai (Dragon's Line). Accordingly, a river was called Shui Long or Water Dragon, indicating the reverence in which water—as a natural element—was held.

The ideal site for a human construction, such as a city, village, palace, mansion, or tomb, was thought to be one where the site was in balance with the surrounding mountains and rivers. For a house, this would mean that the Dragon's Line was behind the building, a lake or curving river was some distance to the front, and protective hills were placed to the left and right.

In China, the dragon represents primal power. The land is said to be crossed by paths of energy, the "Dragons' Lines." The mountains and rivers are believed to have living spirits.

Another Feng Shui model identifies each of the four directions surrounding a site with an animal. At the back is the Black Turtle, which conveys stability and security from attack. To the front is the Red Phoenix, which represents open vision and the collation of information. The Green Dragon, to the left of the site, and the White Tiger, to the right, represent privacy and protection. Together these creatures are known as the Four Spirits. They are linked to the four seasons and the four cardinal points.

The animal spirits can also be connected with the elements through the colors that they represent. In this case a fifth animal spirit is included in the model and is placed at the center of the site. The Yellow Snake is protected the other four spirits and represents the ideal Feng Shui location.

HOME AND BUSINESS FENG SHUI

In the past, Feng Shui was divided into two categories. One deals with the Yin Zhai or tombs, and the other deals with Yang Zhai or the dwellings of the living. Today, much less emphasis is given to finding propitious burial sites, but Feng Shui can still be divided into two categories: residential (Yin) and business (Yang).

For residential Feng Shui, we are mainly looking for a place that is good for our private family life and good for our health. We are looking for somewhere peaceful, private, and convenient for us in every way. The internal arrangements of every room in the house should also be favorable in all aspects.

However, if we are looking at the Feng Shui for a business or an office, we will be looking for a place where there is a more active environment. Here a more open aspect and proximity to other business premises are important factors. Such a place should reflect our social and career aspirations.

If we were to choose a house for our home by a traffic circle, it would not normally be considered good Feng Shui. However, for a store or a café this site could be ideal. If we put a desk in our private home facing the garden with our backs to the wall where the door is, we could feel perfectly comfortable. Yet if we did the same in an office, turning our backs on the direction from where our business colleagues or customers would appear, it would be considered quite inappropriate.

Increasingly, Feng Shui experts are being hired by both private individuals and big businesses to harmonize the energy in a building. Their suggestions may include structural changes, rearranging the furniture, adding or removing plants and mirrors, and painting a room a different color. Because the energy is subtle, Feng Shui works on a sliding scale; few buildings are in complete harmony with their surroundings. The energy in most Western homes and offices can be improved cheaply or at no expense at all (just moving a wastepaper basket can make a difference), but large-scale changes can be costly.

Though the concept and practice of Feng Shui is deeply rooted in the Chinese esoteric tradition, the real value of it goes beyond cultural barriers. Environmental consciousness has greatly increased in the West in the last two decades. This in turn has made people reflect on the effect that their immediate environments—their homes and places of work—can have on their lives.

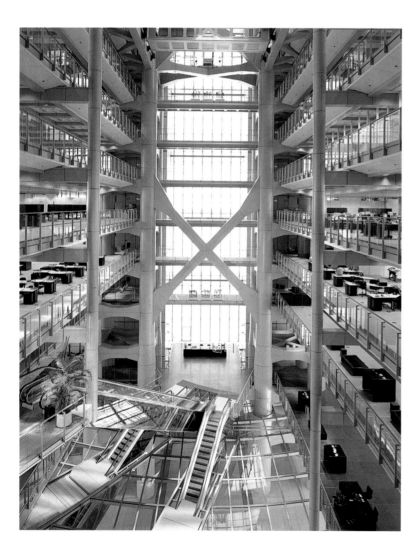

The headquarters of the Hongkong & Shanghai Bank on Hong Kong Island were completed in 1985. During the construction of this ultra-modern building, the Western architects, Foster Associates, consulted a Feng Shui master to ensure that its exterior was in harmony with the cityscape, and that its interior was a propitious workspace.

FENG SHUI IN THE HOME AND AT THE OFFICE

One of the most important functions of home Feng Shui is to place the bed in the right position. Equivalent importance is given in office Feng Shui to the positioning of the desk and the chair. A well-situated bed will promote good health and a happy family relationship, while a properly placed desk and chair will bring good fortune and success.

Simply speaking, a bed should not be exposed to the draft between the door and the window, or too near to the door or the window if possible. It should have a good sense of security and coziness. From your bed you should be able to see people coming in to the room and not be seen easily from the door by people passing or entering.

Similarly, an office desk and chair should be in a position where the person working should be backed by a wall with an open view in the front. It is not recommended to have the chair at the desk facing a wall with the person's back exposed to the door. A chair backed by the window is also not ideal.

When buying or building a house, we should first decide on the area in which we want to live in, whether it is to be in the country or in the city. Then we should be aware of which direction the house should face, taking into account its surroundings. When we have found a property, we need to consider whether it is suitable for us (the family) to live in. We need to check its structure and decide which room is to be used for what purpose. Any structural flaws will have to be addressed and rooms redecorated if they are not in line with Feng Shui principles. Finally, we should decide the date and time to commence building or moving in or out of the house.

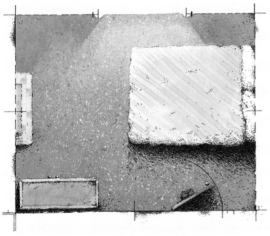
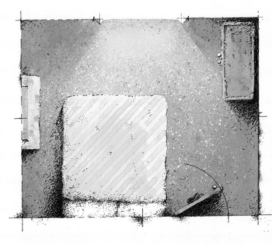

The bed's position in the room on the left is not good. It is in the energy path flowing between the door and window. Those passing would be able to see the bed if the door was ajar. The position of the bed in the room on the right is much better as it offers more privacy and security.

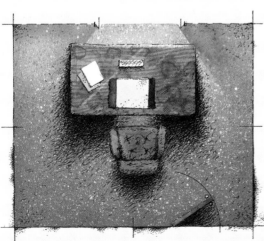
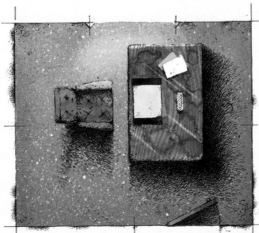

The position of the desk in the left picture means that a worker has his or her back to anyone entering the room, which makes him or her seem both vulnerable and rude. The energy in the office to the right is much better, because people are seen as they enter.

ENERGIZING YOUR ENVIRONMENT

Our home environment both reflects and affects the state of our energy. A number of things can be done to increase the harmony and energy flow of our homes, without enormous expenditure. Try to avoid clutter, which can reflect a cluttered mind. Clearing closets and drawers of unwanted clothes and bric-a-brac can leave us feeling physically and emotionally lighter, and create space for new energy to enter.

Color and light affect us not just through the eyes: colors (like sounds) vibrate at particular frequencies that subtly affect our physical and energy well-being. In the home, certain colors are conducive to particular activities. Pink encourages calm, peace of mind, and loving qualities, and is good for bedrooms and children's rooms. Blue is also peaceful, though less warm for bedrooms. Yellow encourages intellectual activities. Green is restful and healing, good for living and dining rooms. Red leads to an increase in activity and aggression, so should be used sparingly. Use bright colors in moderation only. This is especially important for children; they love vivid colors, but these should be restricted to toys and clothes; for walls and furnishings they can be over-stimulating.

The color of your clothes and the food that you eat can also affect your mood and personality. People who become angry easily may find they become more calm if they avoid red clothes and red meat, the very things that might benefit a more lethargic person.

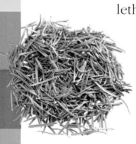

Music is another powerful way of changing a person's mood. Some types of music have been found to be energizing, while others induce calm. Music can also alter a person's state of consciousness.

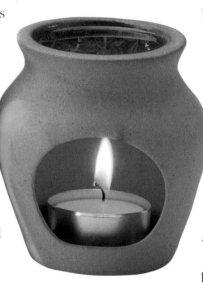

Oil burners work by gently heating an essential oil so that it evaporates. Airborne molecules then enter the body through the lungs.

The quantity and quality of lighting is also important. Avoid fluorescent lights, because they are known to induce headaches in some people. For areas where you read, sew or study, buy full-spectrum light bulbs that have the same quality as daylight.

In recent years, more and more people have developed pollution-related conditions, such as asthma and food allergies. These have a direct link with the rise in number of cars on the road and therefore exhaust fumes. Even indoors we are at risk from pollution, particularly in built-up areas. This can be helped by the use of air filters and ionizers—the latter also counteract the effects of electromagnetic pollution. As electromagnetic beings ourselves, we can be adversely affected by environmental radiation—not only from pylons, which can seriously damage health, but also from computers, mobile phones, television sets, and other types of electronic equipment. Microwave ovens are unlikely to affect us directly but seem to destroy the vitality of food, so should only be used in emergencies. Even electric blankets are best avoided since they generate large electrical fields.

House plants help to keep the atmosphere clean and vital; if you have a word processor, keep plants near by to mop up radiation, particularly at the back of the machine. For the monitor, invest in a protective screen that eliminates electromagnetic transmissions. If you use computers a lot at work, walking among trees will help to restore your energy balance. It also helps to wear clothes made of natural fibers and to wash them daily.

Essential oils are a pleasant way to keep the atmosphere fresh and are helpful for particular moods. Keep a stock of bergamot, camomile, clary sage, lavender, rose, rosemary, sandalwood, and ylang-ylang to infuse in an

CRYSTALS AND THEIR CARE

Energy-conscious people are turning more and more to crystals for healing both living systems and atmospheres. They are believed to enhance and focus healing energy and to have specific healing properties themselves. They can also be used to keep the atmosphere clean, for distant healing, for energizing plants, to counteract electromagnetic pollution, and so on.

There are thousands to choose from, but the most commonly used are quartz (rock crystal), rose quartz, and amethyst. Quartz can be used for general healing and protection purposes; rose quartz enhances love and self-love; and amethyst has spiritual properties—keep one beside you when meditating.

When buying a crystal, make your choice intuitively. Clear your mind and allow yourself to be open to the energy of the crystals. The one that catches your eye will be the one that will help you. Before using it, clean it under running cold water or soak it overnight in a bowl of salt water. Do not wipe it; leave it to dry in sunlight or moonlight.

You can simply place crystals around your home, or you can dedicate them to particular uses. Hold the crystal while in a meditative state, and mentally state your intention for it. Then place it where it's needed—by your word processor, by your bed, or wherever it may be useful.

Crystals will absorb negative vibrations, so remember to cleanse and re-energize them at regular intervals.

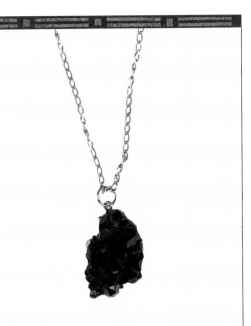

Amethyst crystals have spiritual qualities and so are often used as meditative tools.

oil burner. Fill the top of the oil burner with water and add 3–4 drops of your chosen essential oil. Then light a nightlight under the pot to fill the room with fragrance. Other ways of making the essential oil infuse include: placing a couple of drops on the wick of a candle just before lighting it; adding a few drops to a cup of water beneath a radiator or to a hot, running bath; dripping a small amount onto a light bulb; putting a couple of drops in a water-filled atomizer as a room spray; and adding some to wood before burning it in an open fireplace. Alternatively, you can dissolve the essential oil in a base oil and give yourself or a friend an Aromatherapy massage (see pages 88–91).

You can either use one essential oil at a time or you can combine two or three complementary oils. Bergamot is a cooling oil, which also acts as an insect repellent. Camomile promotes a feeling of relaxation and peace, while clary sage is used to fight depression and tension.

Lavender is an all-purpose oil that emits a pleasant, uplifting aroma. Rose induces a feeling of well-being and happiness. Rosemary has many medicinal qualities. It helps combat infectious illnesses and colds, as well as enhancing memory and concentration. Sandalwood and ylang-ylang have a soothing, calming effect and are also used as aphrodisiacs.

Potpourri is a mixture of dried flower petals and seed heads perfumed by a few drops of essential oil.

CONCLUSION

Your body's energy is a subtle yet powerful force, and one that is crucial to your physical and spiritual well-being. Luckily, you do not always have to be conscious of it or tending it. Looking after your body's energy is like breathing—you do it constantly, regularly, and without thinking. However, if you nurture your energy, you can improve its quality and greatly benefit your vitality.

Through the use of this book you can consciously make energy part of your life. By following some of the exercises routinely you will begin to notice changes in your physical, mental, and emotional well-being. You may feel better able to cope with the physical demands of your life. You may get sudden urges to dance and skip, and your body will feel lighter and free from the stresses that weighed you down. You will have greater concentration at work and be better able to "switch off" during your free time. You may begin to sleep more deeply and wake feeling refreshed and revitalized. As you become more aware of your body's energy, you will feel and understand its ebb and flow more clearly. You will also find that you can nurture those around you by grounding, balancing, and giving them your positive energy.

All matter is made up of energy. It permeates every realm of our existence, unifies the cosmos, and unites every atom in our bodies. Energy in the Solar System guides planets, moons, and stars in a complex and constantly changing dance, controlling their position and orbital movement by intricate cycles of attraction and repulsion. The Sun gives energy to all living things on Earth, and we all respond to changes in its power—hence the number of people who suffer Seasonal Affective Disorder (SAD) during the winter months. The Moon is also a powerful force, influencing both the tides and women's menstrual cycles. You may find that you become more aware of the relationship between your own energy and the energy changes in the Solar System at different times of the year.

There is a subtle, energetic link between every living thing on our planet—it is said that even the flapping of a butterfly's wings creates an energy change that can be felt around the planet. You are part of this delicate, life-giving balance and you can benefit by drawing energy from the natural world. Try to find places from which you can absorb energy, such as historic sites, waterfalls, the huge expanse of the sea, mountain peaks, ancient forests, or the sunshine of your own garden.

This book is an introduction to your body's energy and the many ways it can be cultivated. If you would like to progress further, I would advise you to find an inspiring teacher or therapist to guide you on your path.

The age-old idea that all things are related, that the same energy invigorates everything, has resulted in many depictions of Universal Man. This Tibetan thanka *depicts the correspondences between the human body and the cosmos.*

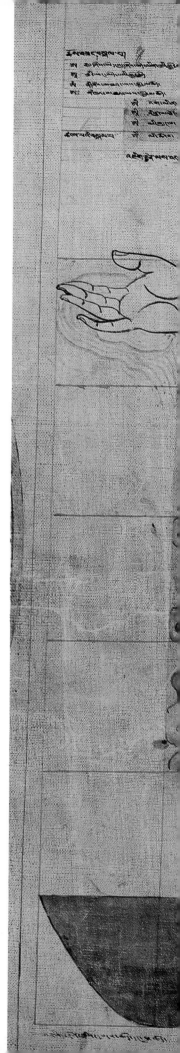

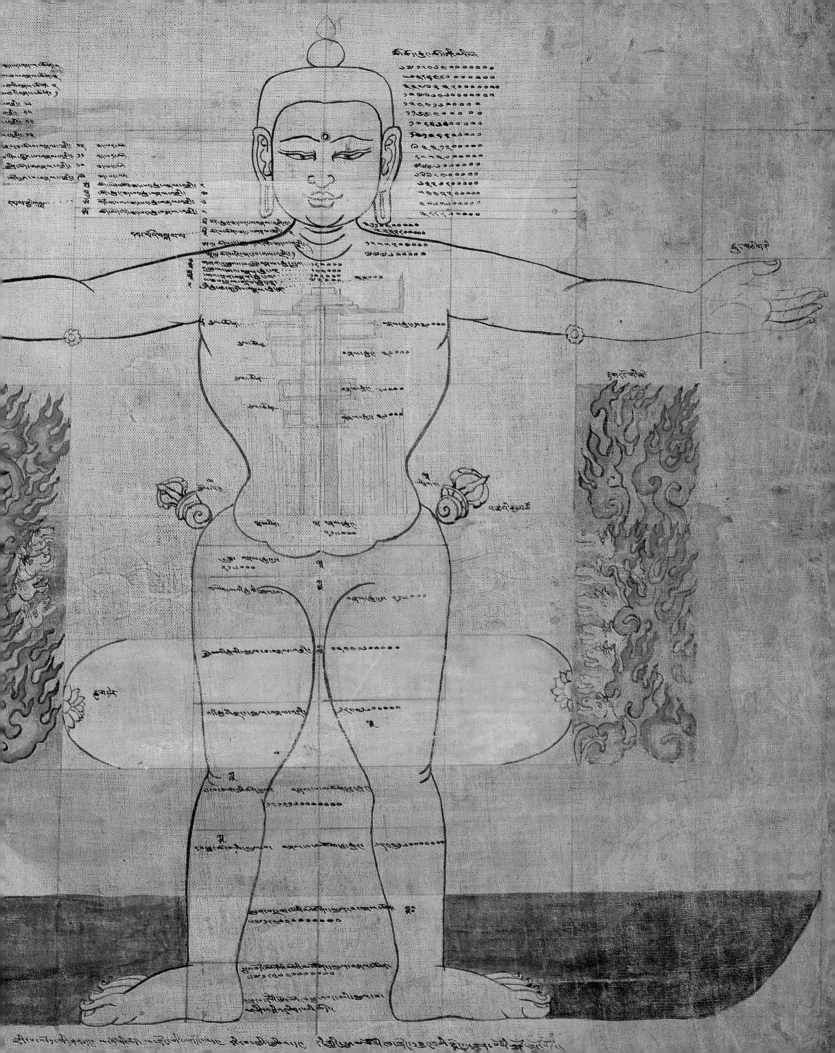

LIST OF CONTRIBUTORS

Carola Beresford-Cooke *(Massage and Aromatherapy)*
A Shiatsu practitioner since 1978, Carola Beresford-Cooke is a founder-member of the Shiatsu Society. She presented a six-part series for Thames Television to accompany her best-seller *Massage for Healing and Relaxation*. She has written and co-written several other books, including *The Book of Massage* and *Acupressure*. She teaches her own techniques at the Institute of Traditional Herbal Medicine and Aromatherapy. Carola Beresford-Cooke is a founding principal of the Shiatsu College, established in 1986. She also holds qualifications in Acupuncture, Acupressure, and Herbal Medicine.

Anthea Courtenay *(Holistic Healing, Posture and Movement, Relaxation, Sleep, and Rest)*
A freelance journalist and writer specializing in complementary medicine, psychology, and healing. Her books include *Natural Sleep, Healing Now, Chiropractic, Your Spine and Your Health*, and *Thorsons Principles of Kinesiology* (with Maggie la Tourelle). She has contributed articles to numerous British publications including *The Guardian, Time Out, Good Housekeeping, The Journal of Alternative Health and Complementary Medicine, Here's Health*, and *The Complete Family Guide to Alternative Medicine*.

Om Prakash Dewan *(Yoga)*
Born and brought up in India, Om Prakash Dewan is a highly qualified Yoga instructor who has taught in London since 1980. He teaches Hatha and Raja Yoga, *pranayama*, chakra meditation, and stress management at London colleges and the Institute of Indian Culture. He has the British Wheel of Yoga Teacher's Diploma and the Advanced Yoga Teacher's Certificate from the International Sivananda Yoga Vedanta School in India. He is also qualified in a wide range of other subjects associated with Alternative Therapies such as Massage, Color Healing, Reflexology, and Counseling.

Dr Shantha Godagama *(Ayurveda)*
Dr Shantha Godagama is one of the world's leading Ayurveda practitioners. He studied Ayurvedic and conventional medicine at Colombo University, Sri Lanka, and also specializes in Acupuncture and Homeopathy. Dr Godagama has worked in Britain since 1979, most recently as a consultant at the prestigious Hale Clinic; he is the Founder President of the Ayurvedic Medical Association U.K. Dr Godagama has presented papers at several international conferences on complementary medicine, and was awarded the Dag Hammarsk Jold Award for Alternative Medicine in 1978.

Emma Mitchell *(Reflexology, Introduction, and Conclusion)*
Emma Mitchell is a qualified Aromatherapist and Reflexologist who has recently opened her own clinic near Winchester, England. She has also studied Kinesiology, Polarity Theory, Nutrition,

Homeopathy, Massage, and Iridology at the Raworth Centre in Dorking, Surrey. Her own interest in health and complementary medicine began with her battle against Hodgkin's Disease, a cancer of the immune system, during which she experienced both chemotherapy and radiotherapy but also gained firsthand awareness of the benefits of meditation and complementary methods of treatment. She is now married with a young daughter and son.

Karen Smith *(Dance)*
A former dancer with the Royal Ballet, Karen Smith became interested in complementary medicine following a car accident that ended her dancing career. During her recovery from paralysis, she received the benefits of Acupuncture, Aromatherapy, Osteopathy, and Reflexology, and subsequently undertook a three-year period of study in complementary medicine, anatomy, and physiology. She is a professionally qualified Reflexologist, Masseuse, and Aromatherapist, and runs a successful clinic in London.

Maggie la Tourelle *(Kinesiology)*
A Holistic Health therapist, teacher and writer, Maggie la Tourelle has taught Kinesiology professionally since 1984. She currently runs training courses in Kinesiology and communication skills. She also holds qualifications in other healing disciplines, including Neuro-Linguistic Programming (NLP), healing, and psychotriciapy. Her previous publications include *Thorsons Principles of Kinesiology* (with Anthea Courtenay).

Zhixing Wang *(Qigong)*
Zhixing Wang is one of the leading Qigong practitioners in the West. He trained under the Chinese Doctor and Daoist Master Jiang Chang Qing, as well as with two other Qigong masters: Zhang Hong Bao and Yan Xin. Zhixing Wang now runs the Chinese Heritage Ltd, an international organization offering Qigong workshops and retreats, and teaches his personal style of Qigong, known as Hua Gong, in Europe and the USA. He is a consultant at the Hale Clinic in London and has written articles for many complementary health magazines.

Jacqueline Young *(Chinese, Japanese, and Tibetan Ideas of Energy, T'ai Chi, Acupuncture and Acupressure, Eastern Herbal Medicine, Diet, and Ayurvedic nutrition)*
A practitioner and writer specializing in complementary medicine, Jacqueline Young is a member of the British Acupuncture Council and the Guild of Health Writers. She has degrees in psychology, and diplomas in Oriental Medicine and Acupuncture from Tokyo and Beijing. Her previous publications include *Vital Energy, Self-Massage*, and *Acupressure for Health*, and she contributed to *The Complete Family Guide to Alternative Medicine*. Jacqueline Young has practiced martial arts for many years and is a qualified Yoga teacher.

BIBLIOGRAPHY

Acupressure – Jacqueline Young, *Acupressure for Health* (Thorsons, London, 1994).
Chris Jarmey and John Tindall, *Acupressure for Common Ailments* (Gaia Books, London, 1991).

Acupuncture – Peter Firebrace and Sandra Hill, *A Guide to Acupuncture* (Constable, London, 1991).

Alexander Technique – Michael Gelb, *Body Learning* (Aurum Press, London, 1994).

Aromatherapy – Julia Lawless, *Aromatherapy and the Mind* (Thorsons, London, 1994).

Ayurveda – Dr Deepak Chopra, *Return of the Rishi* (Houghton Mifflin Co., USA, 1988).
Dr Deepak Chopra, *Unconditional Life* (Bantam Books, USA, 1992).
Dr Shantha Godagama, *The Handbook of Ayurveda* (Kyle Cathie Ltd, London, 1997).

Chinese Traditional Medicine – Ilza Veith (translation and introductory study) *The Yellow Emperor's Classic of Internal Medicine* (University of California Press, 1972).
Ted Kaptchuk, *The Web that has no Weaver* (Rider, London, 1983).

Do-in – Michio Kushi, *The Book of Do-in* (Japan Publications, Inc., Tokyo and New York, 1979).

Energy Medicine – C. Norman Shealy MD, PhD (Ed.), *The Complete Family Guide to Alernative Medicine* (Element, Shaftesbury, Dorset, 1996).
Dr Richard Gerber, MD, *Vibrational Medicine* (Bear & Co., Santa Fe, New Mexico, USA, 1988).

Flower Remedies – Edward Bach, *Heal Thyself* (C. W. Daniel Co. Ltd, 1931, reprint 1990).
Clare C. Harvey and Amanda Cochrane, *The Encyclopaedia of Flower Remedies* (Thorsons, London, 1995).

Healing – Jack Angelo, *Spiritual Healing, Energy Medicine for Today* (Element, Shaftesbury, Dorset, 1991).
Jack Angelo, *Your Healing Power: A Comprehensive Guide to Channelling Your Healing Energies* (Piatkus Books, London, 1994).
Barbara Ann Brennan, *Hands of Light: A Guide to Healing Through the Human Energy Field* (Bantam Press, London, 1988).
Dolores Krieger, *The Therapeutic Touch: How to use Your Hands to Help or to Heal* (Prentice Hall Inc., 1979).

Homeopathy – Dr Andrew Lockie and Dr Nicola Geddes, *The Complete Guide to Homeopathy* (Dorling Kindersley, London, 1995).
Miranda Castro, *The Complete Homeopathy Handbook* (Macmillan, London, 1990).

Kinesiology – Maggie la Tourelle with Anthea Courtenay, *Principles of Kinesiology* (Thorsons, London, 1997).
John F. Thie, DC, *Touch for Health* (De Vorss & Co., Marina del Rey, California, USA, 1973).

Massage – Julie Henderson, *The Lover Within* (Station Hill Press, 1986).
Lucinda Lidell, et al., *The Book of Massage* (Ebury Press, London, 1984).
John Steele, *Earthmind* (Harper and Row, London, 1989).
Jacqueline Young, *Self-Massage* (Thorsons, London, 1997).

Physical Therapies – Anthea Courtenay, *Chiropractic: Your Spine and Your Health* (Penguin Books, London, 1987).

Polarity Therapy – Franklyn Sills, *The Polarity Process: Energy as a Healing Art* (Element, Shaftesbury, Dorset, 1989).
Randolph Stone, *Polarity Theory* (CRCS Sebastopol, 1986 and 1987).

Qigong – James MacRitchie, *Chi Kung, Cultivating Personal Energy* (Health Essentials, Element, Shaftesbury, Dorset, 1993).
Master Lam Kam Chuen, *The Way of Energy* (Gaia Books Ltd, London, 1991).
Jacqueline Young, *Vital Energy* (Hodder and Stoughton, Sevenoaks, 1990).
Zhixing Wang, *Qigong Video for Healing and Learning* (Chinese Heritage Publications Ltd, London).

Reflexology – Inge Dougans with Suzanne Ellis, *The Art of Reflexology* (Element, Shaftesbury, Dorset, 1992).

Shiatsu – Oliver Cowmeadow, *The Art of Shiatsu* (Element Shaftesbury, Dorset, 1992).
Nigel Dawes, *The Shiatsu Workbook* (Piatkus, London, 1991).

Yoga – B.K.S. Iyengar, *Light on Yoga* (Thorsons / Aquarian Press, London, 1991).
Sivananda Yoga Centre, *The Book of Yoga* (Ebury Press, London, 1983).
Swami Vishnudevananda, *The Complete Illustrated Book of Yoga* (Three Rivers Press, New York, USA, 1988).

USEFUL ADDRESSES

Acupressure
The Acupressure Institute
1533 Shattuck Avenue
Berkeley CA 94709
Tel: (510) 845-1059

Acupuncture
The American Academy of
Medical Acupuncture
5820 Wiltshire Boulevard
Suite 500
Los Angeles CA 90036
Tel: (213) 937-5514

Alexander Technique
North American Society of
Teachers of the Alexander
Technique
PO Box 5536
Playa del Rey CA 90296
Tel: (800) 473-0620

Aromatherapy
Aromatherapy Institute of
Research
PO Box 2354
Fair Oaks CA 95628
Tel: (916) 965-7546

National Association for Holistic
Aromatherapy
219 Carl Street
San Francisco CA 94117
Tel: (415) 564-6799

Ayurveda
The Ayurvedic Institute
11311 Menaud NE, Suite A
Albuquerque NM 87112
Tel: (505) 291-9698

Complementary Medicine
American Holistic Health
Association
PO Box 17400
Anaheim CA 92817-7400
Tel: (714) 779-6152

Flower Remedies
Flower Essence Society
PO Box 459
Nevada City CA 95959
Tel: (916) 265-9163

Homeopathy
American Institute of
Homeopathy
1585 Glencoe
Denver CO 80220
Tel: (303) 370-9164

International Foundation for
Homeopathy
2366 Eastlake Avenue, E, 329
Seattle WA 98102
Tel: (206) 324-8230

Kinesiology
International College of
Applied Kinesiology
PO Box 25276
Shawnee Mission
Kansas 66225-5276
Tel: (913) 648-2828

Touch for Health Foundation
1174 North Lake Avenue
Pasadena CA 91104-3797
Tel: (818) 794-1181

Massage
American Massage Therapy
Association
820 Davis Street, Suite 100
Evanston IL 60201-4444
Tel: (847) 864-0123

Associated Bodywork and
Massage Professionals
28677 Buffalo Park Road
Evergreen CO 80439-7347
Tel: (303) 674-8478

Physical Therapies
American Chiropractic
Association
1701 Clarendon Boulevard
Arlington VA 22209
Tel: (703) 276-8800

American Academy of
Osteopathy
3500 DePauw Boulevard
Suite 1080
Indianapolis IN 46268
Tel: (317) 879-1881

American Polarity Therapy
Association
2888 Bluff Street, Suite 149
Boulder CO 80301
Tel: (303) 545-2080

International Chiropractors
Association
1110 N. Glebe Road, Suite 1000
Arlington VA 22201
Tel: (703) 528-5000

Qigong
Leon Smith
220 Wood Drive
Ancramdale NY 2503
Tel: (518) 329-4521

Reflexology
International Institute of
Reflexology
PO Box 12642
St Petersburg FL 33733-2642
Tel: (813) 343-4811

Reflexology Association of
America
4012 South Rainbow Boulevard
PO Box K-585
Las Vegas NV 89103-2059
Tel: (717) 823-8750

Shiatsu
The American Oriental
Bodywork Therapy Association
6801 Jericho Turnpike
Syosset NY 11791-4413
Tel: (516) 364-5533

Yoga
The International Association of
Yoga Therapists
109 Hillside Avenue
Mill Valley CA 94941
Tel: (415) 381-0876

INDEX

Page numbers in *italic* refer to captions.

ACKNOWLEDGMENTS

The publisher would like to thank the following people, museums, and photographic libraries for permission to reproduce their material. Every care has been taken to trace copyright holders. However, if we have omitted anyone we apologize and will, if informed, make corrections in any future editions.

t: top; c: center; b: bottom; l: left; r: right

Endpapers: Mimi Lipton, Serindia Publications, London; page 10 Science Photo Library; page 11t and b Hutchison Library; page 12 The Vatican Library / Bridgeman Art Library; page 16 Hutchison Library; page 18 Science and Society Picture Library; page 20 Images Colour Library; page 21 Getty Images; page 22 Graham Harrison; page 23t and l The Needham Institute, Cambridge; page 23r Hutchison Library; page 32 Hutchison Library; page 33 Ancient Art and Architecture; page 34t Graham Harrison; page 34b Ancient Art and Architecture; page 36 Science and Society Picture Library; page 40 Mandanjeet Singh; page 42tl British Library (Or 24099); page 42br Images Colour Library; page 43 Images Colour Library; page 44t and b Images Colour Library; page 46 Sam Fogg Rare Books, London; page 56 Graham Harrison; page 58 AKG, London; page 64 Hutchison Library; page 74 British Library / Bridgeman Art Library; page 78 Mary Evans Picture Library; page 88tl British Library (Add. 27255 f.340b); page 88br Ancient Art and Architecture; page 89 DBP Archives; page 89t Serindia Publications, London (plate 54); page 89b Werner Forman Archives; page 92t Michael Holford; page 92b Hutchison Library; page 102 Science and Society Picture Library; page 103 National Palace Museum, Taiwan / Bridgeman Art Library; page 104 British Library; page 106 Zefa; page 107 Life File; page 110 Science Photo Library; page 114 Images Colour Library; page 116 Science Photo Library; page 117t Scala; page 117b DBP Archives; page 118 British Library (Add. 24099 f.118); page 120t British Library (Add. Or 1426); page 120b British Library (Add. 27255 f.274v); page 121 Hutchison Library; page 122 Science and Society Picture Library; page 123 DBP Archives; page 128r Getty Images; page 128l and 129 Naito Museum of Pharmaceutical Science and Industry, Gifu, Japan; page 130 Sam Fogg Rare Books, London; page 131 Getty Images; page 133 Abbas / Magnum Pictures; page 134 Antonio Martinelli; page 135t Pepita Seth; page 135b Mimi Lipton; page 136 AKG, London; page 140 Bridgeman Art Library; page 145 Scala; page 146 Zhang Shui Cheng / Bridgeman Art Library; page 147 Images Colour Library; page 148 Richard Bryant / Arcaid; page 152 Mimi Lipton.

All commissioned photography by Antonia Deutsch.

Chair provided by Habitat.

Principle illustrations by Elaine Cox: pages 4/5, 8/9, 14/15, 38/39, 54/55, 76/77, 100/101, 124/125
Additional illustrations by: David Atkinson page 151; Hannah Fermin page 1; Tony Lodge pages 18, 19, 36, 93, 111

The publisher would like to thank Liz Cowen, Mike Darton, and Margaret Miller for their contributions to this book. Also, Sam Fogg Rare Books, London, the Needham Institute, Cambridge, and Serindia Publications, London for their help in researching the subject.

Emma Mitchell would particularly like to thank Daphne Clark, Pat Essex, Alickie Gravel, Caroline Jory, Helen Merfield, Alex Mitchell, Georgie Ruthven, and all the teachers at the Raworth Centre, Dorking for their support and inspiration.

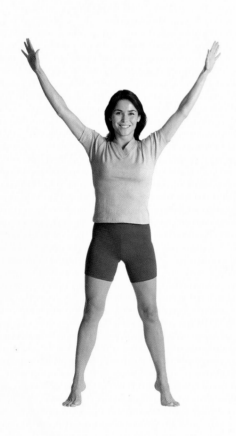